The Missing Medical Text

The Missing Medical Text

HUMANE PATIENT CARE

ANTHONY R. MOORE
M.B., M.S. (Melb.), F.R.A.C.S.,
B.A. (Cantab.)

Senior Lecturer in Surgery,
University of Melbourne
Surgeon, Royal Melbourne Hospital
Surgeon, Mount Royal Hospital for the Aged

MELBOURNE UNIVERSITY PRESS

1978

First published 1978

Printed in Australia by
Wilke and Company Limited, Clayton, Victoria 3168, for
Melbourne University Press, Carlton, Victoria 3053
U.S.A. and Canada: International Scholarly Book Service, Inc.,
Box 555, Forest Grove, Oregon 97116
Great Britain, Europe, the Middle East, Africa and the Caribbean:
International Book Distributors Ltd (Prentice-Hall International),
66 Wood Lane End, Hemel Hempstead, Hertfordshire HP2 4RG England

National Library of Australia Cataloguing in Publication data

Moore, Anthony Robert, 1940-
The missing medical text
ISBN 0 522 84139 2
1. Social medicine. 2. Medicine. I. Title.
301.5

To music

the infinite therapy

CONTENTS

PREFACE

There is something sinister about present-day medical education. In this book I have tried to identify what is wrong and offer a solution. The book has been written for all people concerned with humane health care, and their patients. In fact, the book has been 'written' partly by medical students, for much of the text is made up of their contributions to a series of round-table discussions which took place while they were attending my course in medical humanities.

Before outlining the details of that course, and before revealing the students' comments during the discussions, I would like to explain why the course was created.

Over recent years there has been a gradual but significant increase in public criticism of the medical profession. I have been gravely concerned about the slow erosion of public regard for doctors, and believe that the fragmentation of the warmth and favour in which we are held by our patients will gradually undermine the finer aspects of our doctorship. As the medical profession has been a treasury of so many of the traditional qualities of social virtue, our public standing should be one of excellence. The long list of these qualities–pity, compassion, charity, concern, selflessness, applied scientific intelligence, social responsibility, and human sensitivity–should guarantee public regard. If it does not, something is desperately wrong; for an unreserved affection for those who relieve the suffering of others has been an uncontested sentiment in almost all societies. Therefore, in any age, the natural attitude of the public towards its medical profession should be one of warmth, regard, and respect. If public opinion or social sentiment expresses antagonism rather than affection, the profession should heed the warning by 'healing itself' before presuming on the prejudices of commentators or the ignorance of the public. As a profession we must be vigilant against anything which can be interpreted as professional arrogance, indifference, or isolation. The public notices everything, and lasting dislike is often a consequence of occasional disgust.

I believe most of the present criticism levelled at the medical profession is valid. But I also believe that much of it could have been avoided. Many of our professional blemishes arise as a result of the way medical students are educated, or from the example they are shown by those who were educated in the same mould before them.

In an attempt to redress some of the imbalances in medical education I have designed a short course called Medical Humanities which is concerned with the *art* of medicine rather than its *science*.

I view this book as a journey in partnership in which the writer and reader clasp hands to aid each other over difficult terrains and to show each other new views. I invite the reader to join in this exploration rather than to rest in the docile reception of ideas stated dogmatically. The questions implied in these chapters are not posed for an argumentative victory, but rather to bring forward themes for discussion. They are not attempts to show whether or not on a certain issue my opinion or the students' view is correct, but to gain agreement that the problem is worthy of discussion.

Although this book challenges medical students and the way they are educated, the issues considered are relevant for everyone involved with health care, and all those who, like me, struggle to appreciate the wonderful complexities of human nature.

I have suggested that this book is concerned with the delicate area of medical practice which is loosely called the art of medicine. Let us therefore begin with a consideration of what medicine as an art means.

ACKNOWLEDGEMENTS

There is no way I can adequately thank the students

Doctor Theodore Redpath
Trinity College, University of Cambridge
whose teaching example was an inspiration

Professor Maurice Ewing
University of Melbourne
who provided the encouragement and opportunity

Mrs Margaret Best
my secretary, whose loyalty and labour is boundless

Judy Share
my assistant, for her care and calmness

Sandra
my wife, for believing

THE ART OF MEDICINE[1]

Dr Lydgate carried the conviction that the medical profession as it might be *was the finest in the world; presenting the most perfect interchange between science and art; offering the most direct alliance between intellectual conquest and social good.*[2]

George Eliot

What then does the art of medicine mean? Do we have a clear concept of its essence and relevance, or is there just a vague sense of concession towards something which is acknowledged in theory—or when one is teaching students or nurses—but ignored in the clinic or ward? Does mention of it produce a flutter of embarrassment or even hostility from doctors because, like a confession of our personal deficiencies, it is unmanly and should not be dwelt on or discussed? I believe that the old definition of the art of medicine (a practical knowledge of the techniques of history-taking, physical examination, and therapeutics) is no longer helpful because it has become incorporated into the scientific medical method.

In present practice the art of medicine seems to exist as a rather indefinite and ephemeral thing—a cloud which covers the strata of medical practice above the sharp, sure peaks of science. It is a mist which drifts in an atmosphere 'outside the scope of this particular work' or which is carried by crosscurrents away from 'further discussion in relation to that particular topic': a cumulus medicus unindexed. Yet the profession wrinkles and dies without it; for as science is the soil of practice, the art of medicine is its irrigation.

It is difficult to define precisely the nature and domain of what I believe to be the art of medicine. But let me try. Much of medical practice rests on scientific truths tested experimentally and monitored clinically. Other areas, like the routines in a clinic or ward, depend on common sense, rules of thumb, and accepted conventions. Beyond these is that area of human conviction where proof is not the ultimate warrant of truth, but where intuition, imagination, tradition, feeling, and sentiment are the foundations of belief. To this world belongs everything about which civilized man cares most. It includes ethics, morals, religion, and aesthetics. It covers discussions of liberty, nationality, justice, love, truth, faith, and knowledge. This is the area of medicine as an art. Its discussions differ from scientific arguments most markedly in this: that even before a debate has begun there is mutual acknowledgement that, in the end, variant opinions are equally valid and equally right for those who hold them. It involves a mutual exploration of a topic rather than a 'talk for triumph' where one disputant is humbled by something of statistical significance or by the authority of an experimental method. Anton Chekhov, physician, playwright, and story-teller, was aware of the dangers: he warned against doctors who are 'completely ignorant of the doubts and disappointments that turn talented men grey', and who are 'firmly convinced that medicine is the best science, that doctors are the best people, and that medical traditions are the best traditions?'[3]

There are, therefore, two important principles to acknowledge. The first is that the art of medicine depends on a different form of thought compared with its science—one which is similar to that which we use to assess a moral position, a painting, or a poem. The second, which follows from the first, is that the conclusions developed are problematical, or open to question.

I believe that for most medical students there is nothing in their selection, their curricula, or the example they are shown by senior colleagues, which stimulates them to acknowledge and explore the territory of the art of medicine. Without any sense of betrayal towards my senior colleagues, I must confess that the defects of the young become the deformities of the old.

As a result of this deficiency we lose much. For the art of medicine determines just when experimental objectivity becomes human insensitivity. It judges at which point clinical busyness causes the patient's concerns to be dismissed. It warns when scientific certainty becomes professional arrogance, and when tiredness becomes the excuse for intolerance. The art of medicine helps prevent devaluation of the uncommunicative or irritating patient, and, most importantly, it harmonizes public accountability with professional allegiance.

The art of medicine stimulates the attitude of mind which concedes that on certain issues the patient knows what is right for him or her, and the public senses what is best for it. Not because they are right, but because on these issues there is no absolute *right*. Charles Kingsley, in his novel about the cholera epidemic of the early 1850s, warned his doctor hero:

> Every fresh specimen of humanity which he examined was so much gained in general knowledge. Very true, Thomas Thurnall; provided the method be the sound and deep one, which will lead you down in each case to the real living heart of humanity; but what if your method be altogether a shallow and cynical one, ... grounded not on faith and love for human beings, but on something very like suspicion and contempt? You will be but too likely, doctor,

> to make the coarsest mistakes . . . [for] there are more things, not only in heaven, but in the earthiest of earth, than are dreamt of in your philosophy.[4]

Doctors and nurses are practical people. The end point of their vocational efforts is usually tangible and immediate. It is not easy for doctors to cast off the securities offered by science, for the demands of diagnosis do not tolerate error, and the practical consequences of therapy give little margin for mistake. Everything in our training reinforces the importance of achieving accuracy in clinical decisions; and for the part of medical practice under the realm of science this must always be so.

But all attitudes and methods have their limits, and to highlight their shortcomings does *not* imply criticism of their efficiencies. Professions tend to be right in what they affirm, and wrong in what they ignore. Medical education today seems to deny that, at its foundation, the profession rests on a knowledge and understanding of human nature. With its affections, convictions, whims, and sentiments, human nature is anything but a science. The nature of man is intricate; and the objects of his concern—his social beliefs, his behaviour patterns, and his fears and fantasies—are of the greatest possible complexity. Therefore no simple attitude or view, be it scientific or legalistic, can be put forward as a tidy code of what is acceptable or expected in human behaviour.

How much concession is made to the non-scientific aspects of patient care in medical education? Garrison, the medical historian, made a plea that 'the real student of medicine will see his Hippocrates as he does his Homer, his Harvey as he does his Shakespeare, and his Sydenham as he does his Milton'.[5] Unfortunately and ironically his wish is realized—for they are neglected equally.

Sir William Osler, the physician and medical philosopher, expressed concern that 'by the neglect of studies of the humanities, which has been too general, the profession loses a very precious quality'.[6] He recommended ten books for the bedside of the doctor. Apart from saying that the list is a little light on poets and quite substantial on Christians and stoics, I have no hesitation in agreeing with him. The books he suggested were: the Old and New Testaments, Shakespeare's *Works*, Montaigne's *Essays*, Plutarch's *Lives*, Marcus Aurelius's *Meditations*, Epictetus, Thomas Browne's *Religio Medici*, Cervantes' *Don Quixote*, Emerson's *Essays*, and the writings of O. W. Holmes. If one was to try to 'modernize' the list one could suggest the writings of Charles Dickens, Fielding's *Tom Jones*, George Eliot's *Middlemarch*, Lewis's *Arrowsmith*, and Camus's *The Outsider*.

The singularity of the scientific approach in medicine had its origins in the understandably drastic revision of the medical school curricula in the 1850s. Practical ideals led educational zealots to cut from the syllabus all subjects which were not directly applicable to the treatment of disease. In a speech to the Americans called 'Literature and Science', Matthew Arnold, the Victorian poet, critic, and scholar, captured this attitude:

> The usual education in the past has been mainly literary. The question is, whether the studies which were long supposed to be best for all of us are practically the best now; . . . the tyranny of the past, many think, weighs injuriously on the predominance given to letters in education. The question is raised whether, to meet the needs of modern life, the predominance ought not now to pass from letters to science . . .[7]

And my question is: 'ought not now' the predominance to pass a little in the opposite direction? While I agree with Professor T. H. Huxley, surgeon and scholar, that 'for the purpose of attaining real culture, an exclusively scientific education is at least as effectual as an exclusively literary education',[8] I am moved without timidity to suggest that the ultimate efficacy of either *exclusively* is meagre. The disproportion, the imbalance, and the heaviness, is now in favour of science in medical education. It is now that we need the yeast of the humanities to leaven the dough in medicine—for without it we shall grow stale and the public will murmur about our mould.

How can we restore the balance? I know that medical school curricula are full, and that students and doctors are too busy and too tired to grapple with the musings of some ancient, or the aesthetics of 'sweetness and light'. Perhaps; perhaps we are too busy making and remaking the rails on which the profession shunts, without the time, money or interest, to construct the signals of safety or the points which provide the scenic route.

Go into the medical libraries and look at the books and journals. Take up the medical syllabus and observe the subjects. Gaze at our research grants and note their distribution. Then pause—and judge how great is the writing, time, and money spent on medicine as a science, and how mean is that given to medicine as an art. Then go into the wards and clinics and see the *human* problems we are asked to cope with. Our priorities are exclusive. Our product is pure line but lacks hybrid vigour.

It is one thing to criticize, but what can be done to try to reduce the imbalance? What can we do to restore a sense of proportion? I believe there is an easy, efficient, and inexpensive way to aid the art of medicine: the introduction of studies in medical humanities. Such a faculty should draw on literature, art, and the classics for examples that reveal the complexities of human action, and the difficulties of human communication. It should look to philosophy for the study of ethical systems and the tradition of philosophical thought. It should help doctors with their own human dilemmas, and aid them in the understanding of the paradoxes at play in their patients. It should stimulate critical questioning of all dogma. It should not indoctrinate but scrutinize all doctrines.

Goethe, who was an oak of a man, was someone who transcended the boundaries of art and science:

> It causes us so agreeable a sensation to occupy ourselves with what we can half do, that no person ought to find fault with the dillettante, when he is spending his time over an art which he can never learn; nor blame the artist if he chooses to pass over the border of his own art, and amuse himself in some neighbouring field.[9]

As medical men and women we must not be frightened to trespass on the territories of our colleagues in the arts. They may wince at our indelicate interpretations and smile at our lack of eloquence and elegance. Yet our opportunity for the everyday application of the essence of their subjects is unequalled.

There will be some who criticize the artificiality of the separation between medicine as an art and science—who will stress that they are mutually interdependent. I agree with them. I agree that when the practice of medicine functions *successfully and harmoniously* its art and science do not merely coexist, they coalesce; as with any fertilization where two different elements fuse to form a new viable entity. There will be some who will question the whole concept of the ability to educate for attitudes of mind, and I agree with them, it is difficult. Teacher performance is a greater guide to students than teacher precept. There will be others who will say it is too difficult to do. I have nothing to say to them, but Shelley has: 'A thing is good in that it tends to produce that which though impossible, yet were it possible, would be desirable.'[10]

It is my belief that if the art of medicine is allowed to wander weakly over a cliff, the science of medicine, with all its power, will not abolish gravity. And it was from fear that medical students are given no opportunity formally to consider the area of the art of medicine during their studies that I created the Medical Humanities course.

THE MEDICAL HUMANITIES COURSE

It is uncomfortable to see how meagre is the cultural baggage, how callow the manners, how unexercised the imagination and sympathies of our medical students must remain unless we open them to the resources of Humanism . . . How can we expect such a one to have the valences that will enable him to combine effectively with patients in the bewilderment and loneliness and anxieties of illness.[1]

Alan Gregg

In a medical school it is difficult to provide an opportunity for discussion of the broader cultural, philosophical, and human issues which are relevant to doctorship. Time, utilitarian demands, faculty requirements, and the 'scientific-objective' approach all conspire to subvert the ideal of a general education for doctors. In particular, it is a delicate task to create an environment where the students take the intellectual initiative in a consideration of human issues.

In an attempt to provide such an opportunity, I have designed a short course which is structured around a consideration of extracts from classic literary works. Many perceptive and sensitive writers in literature have captured several of the most delicate and difficult tasks of doctorship. I believe there are lessons in their works–lessons which we cannot learn anywhere else with ease–which all members of the medical profession need to consider. With this in mind I made a selection of about eighty short extracts from the pages of literature, philosophy, and history, all of which are relevant to medicine. They allude either to the experience of being a patient, to the doctor's performance, or to professional behaviour.

Over the past two years all of the students in their first clinical year at the Royal Melbourne Hospital have accepted the challenge of the course. They were the students rostered for formal surgical teaching–a responsibility in which I shared–but their subject for the round-table sessions was something quite different.

Each student was asked to study a number of passages selected from literary works. The students had no prior knowledge of the passages, but were aware of the topic. No pre-session reading was required. The first week, for example, the topic was 'The Patient's Experience of Illness', and included extracts from the following:

'The Convalescent' (1820–33), Charles Lamb
'On Being Ill' (1949), Virginia Woolf
The Magic Mountain (1924), Thomas Mann
War and Peace (1868–9), Leo Tolstoy
The Immoralist (1902), Andre Gide
Cancer Ward (1968), Alexander Solzhenitsyn
Mary Barton (1848), Elizabeth Gaskell
Confessions of an English Opium Eater (1822), Thomas de Quincey
The Bell Jar (1964), Sylvia Plath
Brian's Wife, Jenny's Mum (1975), Gwen Wesson

After the students had studied the list, they indicated to me, as their chairman, which extract they would like to consider first, and then undertook a silent reading for a few minutes. We tried not to rush things too much, but the students indicated they often wanted more time than my eagerness would allow.

When the reading was finished I would open the discussion with a question such as 'What does the passage say?'; 'Do you like or dislike the opinions or characters?'; 'Is the passage true to human experience?'; 'What do you think of the writing?'; and 'What message is there in the extract for us to take back to the ward or clinic?' When the discussion on any passage was finished the group would move on to another, considering only as many in our two-hour session as were compatible with unhurried discussion.

For the last half-hour of each session, portraits and paintings by artists of all centuries, which were relevant to the topic under discussion, were projected as slides and discussed in the same fashion. For a number of practical reasons, the art section will not be presented in this book.

For each of the sessions the form was the same, and the topics we considered during each six-week course were:

1. The Patient's Experience of Illness
2. The Relatives' Experience of Illness
3. Portraits of Doctors in Literature: The Demands of Doctorship
4. The Ethical Landscape
5. Hindrances to Communication: The Patient's Expectations
6. Public Regard for Professional Performance–Past and Present

I selected these topics to try to cover the widest possible range of human medical issues for which appropriate literary extracts were available, and to achieve the objectives of the course. They were only 'starting' topics; I do not regard them as important as the topics which grew spontaneously out of the student discussions. And I certainly do not claim that we have considered all the topics which could assist our objectives.

The single most important objective of the course was to allow easy and free-ranging discussions that stimulated the students' intellectual initiatives and encouraged them to formulate and articulate their own point of view. The specific objectives were:

1. To offer a forum for the discussion of aspects of doctorship which are untended in the formal syllabus (83 per cent of the 150 students who have taken the course so far felt that the course stimulated them to consider previously neglected medical topics).

2. To draw on the medical heritage which is recorded in literature, social history, and philosophy (86 per cent indicated that the course contributed to their understanding of the traditions of the medical profession).

3. To assist the ideal of cultural scope in medical education (two-thirds of the students were stimulated, either frequently or occasionally, to read the books from which the extracts were taken, and this during the six weeks of the course).

4. To heighten sensibility for patient care, and professional self-assessment (83 per cent of the students felt the course contributed to their human understanding in the ward).

5. To expose students to well-written 'non-medical' English.

6. To explore non-scientific ways of thinking and their importance in the consideration of human issues.

On the completion of the course each student anonymously filled out a questionnaire which probed his or her satisfaction with the form and content of the course and with the chairman's performance, and made an assessment of the objectives.

The experience of the course was completely new to the students. Most arrived not knowing what to expect or what was expected of them. For one group of fourteen students all the sessions were tape-recorded. The remainder of the book is made up of the transcripts of those sessions, and records the students' response to the literary passages which were considered. Through their comments I hope you will come to know the students and value their efforts as much as I do. The group recorded was not specially selected, but good fortune would have it that they were special. With each session their performance became more and more distinguished.

To create some variety I have supplemented the transcripts of each week's sessions with six short essays of my own, all of which are relevant to the general theme of the art of medicine.

The sessions were not just a pleasant Friday afternoon chat. They were vigorous and purposeful, usually stimulating and exhausting, occasionally humorous and hostile, and always productive. Here they are.

SESSION 1

THE PATIENT'S EXPERIENCE OF ILLNESS

Chairman: It's always exciting to start with a new group. Could I say 'welcome' and begin. Looking at the reference list, does anyone see a passage that they would like to consider first?

Brendan: Yes; let's start with the passage from Alexander Solzhenitsyn's novel, *Cancer Ward.*

> Within a few hours, that first evening in the ward, Pavel Nikolayevich became haunted with fear.
>
> The hard lump of his tumour—unexpected, meaningless and quite without use—had dragged him in like a fish on a hook and flung him on to his iron bed—a narrow, mean bed, with creaking springs and an apology for a mattress. Having once undressed under the stairs, said good-bye to the family and come up to the ward, you felt the door to all your past life had been slammed behind you, and the life here was so vile that it frightened you more than the actual tumour. He could no longer choose something pleasant or soothing to look at; he had to look at the eight abject beings who were now his 'equals', eight sick men in faded, worn, pink-and-white pyjamas, patched and torn here and there and almost all the wrong size. And he could not even choose what to listen to; he had to listen to these uncultured creatures and their wearisome conversations which had nothing to do with him and were of no interest to him. He would have loved to command them all to be quiet, especially the tiresome fox-haired one with the bandage-grip round his neck and the constricted head. Everyone called him simply 'Yefrem', even though he was not a young man.
> . . .
>
> He needed support, but instead he was being pushed down into a pit. In a matter of hours he had as good as lost all his personal status, reputation and plans for the future—and had turned into eleven stones of hot, white flesh that did not know what tomorrow would bring.[1]

Chairman: Who would like to help us interpret this passage?

David: I think it describes the depersonalization of coming into hospital. It's pretty much applicable to every patient I would have thought. Obviously the situation in our hospital is somewhat less, I mean the comforts are somewhat better in our hospital than in the hospital described, but the human experience of having so many things stripped away from you and being turned into an anonymous sort of nothing is relevant.

Robert: The bit about the pyjamas is good. You know, even in our hospital they take your clothes, put them in a little drawer, and everyone gets pyjamas which are virtually the same. All the sheets are the same, all the bedcovers are the same, all the beds are the same.

Brendan: Yes; the experience comes to a head in the last paragraph when it says 'He needed support, but instead he was being pushed down into a pit. In a matter of hours he had as good as lost all his personal status, reputation and plans for the future'.

Hilary: It also says that he's more worried about being put into hospital than he is about the actual tumour. He's more concerned about what has happened to him—the fact that he has been taken away from his normal surroundings.

Colin: But he is concerned about the tumour as well, because it was the tumour that dragged him and threw him on to the bed. He is not just concerned about his comforts. There is another aspect to the depersonalization.

Rod: Another thing that it says is that dying patients are dragged into hospital. He is brought in and there is nothing that can really be done for him; they run tests, but really nothing is done. They end up staying in a month or so gradually dying in an unfamiliar atmosphere, whereas if they were at home exactly the same thing would happen to them, they would die just as quickly and just as well, but in normal surroundings.

Chairman: What other things are being said in this passage?

Doug: The whole thing sounds just like a punishment. It's just like a prison.

Gillian: I don't think the patient can quite understand why it is happening to him, it's almost as though he was saying, 'Why me?'

Brendan: He's also been removed from all of his peers and friends and mixed up with a lot of people who he thinks are not as good as he is.

Gillian: Yes, he thinks he's better.

Chairman: How did you respond to that Gillian? How did you feel about him feeling better than other patients?

[*A pause.*]

Gillian: I think it makes you less sympathetic towards him, because I guess we can't see any reason why *he* should feel that he is better.

[*General disagreement.*] Just a minute . . . well, hang on . . . I think that could be quite understandable . . . it could make him less able to relate to other human beings . . . he does say they are uncultured.

Chairman: Are there any circumstances in which his attitude could make you *more* sympathetic towards him?
Robert: Yes. It says here that 'he had to listen to these uncultured creatures and their wearisome conversations'. Well now, say this fellow was a lawyer going into a ward full of bricklayers. The point is just of different people, or different people not being able to relate to each other. Their actual occupation doesn't really matter all that much, I don't think.
Chairman: It would be the same for a bricklayer going into a ward full of lawyers?
Rod: Yes, I agree. Also I think it's just like a person being sent to prison for 'life' joining a whole lot of people who have already been there twenty years. The others have been there too long and they have all been pulled down together. He's come into this ward and he is going to end up the same way, but at the moment he is not at the same stage as they are.
Chairman: I like that point.
Dave: What about somebody who walks into a party where everyone else is drunk. I mean, it's the same thing. The main thing is the difference between one person and everyone else.
Hilary: But he is fighting against that. He doesn't want to join them like somebody coming to a party does. He's fighting against getting caught up with them.
Chairman: A student in another group made a metaphorical reading of this passage. He said the patient saw the ward as an extension of his cancer. It was almost as though the tumour had spread out into the ward.
Students: That's good, that is very good.
Chairman: Is this a good passage? Well written?

[*General comment.*] Yes; yes it's very good.

Chairman: How does the author use words to produce and intensify the effect of what is going on?
David: Some of it is very violent. Things like 'slamming of the door', 'dragged him in'. Things are being done *to* him.
Brendan: Yes, and words like 'unexpected', 'meaningless', and 'quite without use' highlight the degradation.

Hilary: You really sympathize with him in that line, because it is so true.

Rod: I think one of the lines that affected me was 'and he could not choose what to look at'. Once he'd got there his whole life was mapped out for him and he had no choice, not even in what he could look at or listen to.

Chairman: Good. Is the sentiment expressed in this passage true to human experience, or is it overstated? Would most patients feel this? Is there any group of patients for whom this passage would seem meaningless?

Nicholas: If a patient was totally attuned to hospital–a chronic attender coming back repeatedly, for example–he wouldn't feel this.

Liz: Some patients feel quite at home in hospital, they are quite happy to have the company of other people; lonely patients for example.

Robert: Yes, and social admissions. A lot of people we saw in the last medical ward were in there for no other reason than there was just no one to look after them at home.

Liz: But even people who haven't come in for social reasons, provided they haven't got a life-threatening condition, enjoy it. They like talking to everybody and it gives them support.

Chairman: Who is notably absent from this passage who may lend that sort of support?

[*General comment.*] Students can, nurses, doctors, social workers, and even other patients in the ward.

Liz: But this passage is concerned with the first few hours of an admission to hospital, so I guess you wouldn't expect all that much contact from anyone right at the start. When you first come in it is a special time because you are thrown straight into an alien situation and you haven't had time to adapt to the strangeness.

Chairman: Good point Liz.

Robert: Yes, every new situation for a human being produces that response.

Chairman: Even starting a new humanities course?

[*Laughter.*]

Rod: One of the things which makes it sound even more like a prison is in the line 'having once undressed under the stairs, and said good-bye to the family', because when you are separated from the family there is nobody in the ward that you know, there are just the eight men and you.

Chairman: Are there any other comments? [*Pause.*] If not let's go on to consider the Sylvia Plath extract; it's only a short passage and I haven't considered it with a group before; it's one of the new extracts I've added since the last group.

> Later Buddy told me the woman was on a drug that would make her forget she's had any pain and that when she swore and groaned she really didn't know what she was doing because she was in a kind of twilight sleep.
>
> I thought it sounded just like the sort of drug a man would invent. Here was a woman in terrible pain, obviously feeling every bit of it or she wouldn't groan like that, and she would go straight home and start another baby, because the drug would make her forget how bad the pain had been, when all the time, in some secret part of her, that long, blind, doorless and windowless corridor of pain was waiting to open up and shut her in again.[2]

Tony: I think the context of the passage is a woman in childbirth. The narrator in the novel has a boyfriend, Buddy, who is a medical student. He is taking her to watch a woman give birth to a child. She looks at things and sees the degradation that the medical profession has imposed on the woman while giving birth–the way they have her legs in the air, and so on. Any sort of participation in giving birth, any real feeling, is denied her because she is doped up.

Rod: I think Tony must have read the book.

[*Laughter.*]

Chairman: Obviously, if some of us have read the books from which the passages have been taken it really isn't fair on others who haven't. I will ask you just to consider the passage as stated here without any knowledge of context and with no real autobiographical interpretation in terms of our knowledge of the author–unless the group wants to. To be fair to everybody, we should just consider what is on the page, and the meanings we all can extract from the passage.

[*General approval.*]

Stuart: I think this is a reflection on pain. Just interpreting the extract, it seems that the narrator feels that it isn't fair that the patient should undergo a certain traumatic event without experiencing pain. And that–I don't know whether she's trying to be cynical or not, but . . .

Chairman: Well, is the passage cynical?

Stuart: Yes.

Chairman: What is the cynicism being expressed about?

Robert: The use of a drug.

Brendan: Yes; it only achieves a short-term purpose.

Robert: It's also cynical about childbirth. She is saying that if the woman hadn't had the drug, she wouldn't have had another kid.

Hilary: She probably thinks that the woman had a right to understand what's happening to her; to have a full memory of it so she can then make a reasonable decision about whether she wants to go through it again, rather than actually suffering without having any memory of it. . . .

Male student: Is she actually suffering? Is pain . . .

Hilary [*continuing*]: Assuming that the woman is suffering . . .

Rod: If you are lying in the street unconscious and someone comes along and kicks you in the shin, it's not painful.

Hilary: But the narrator is assuming that the woman who is giving birth is suffering pain because she is groaning. We are told that . . .

Rod: But the lady herself isn't feeling pain, so why should you say she is feeling pain.

Male student: Is it a terrible assumption to assume someone's feeling pain because they're groaning?

Rod: Pain's subjective. It is not what *you* think she is feeling that's important, it's what she actually feels.

Hilary [*persisting*]: If she's groaning, it must be for some reason.

Stuart: I think it is just like pithing a toad. You look at it and it's wriggling around and you think 'you poor thing', but it's not really feeling any pain.

Chairman: So is having a baby like pithing a toad? Is the pain of childbirth a bad example of the problem of pain in clinical practice?

Liz: I think the pain of childbirth *is* a bad example in that women are much more likely to accept the pain of childbirth as opposed to pain induced by trauma or any other disease. It's something that they have undertaken.

Chairman: Would the sentiment expressed in this passage be out of keeping with the view of the majority of women?

Male student: Yes.

Jane: I think that is the point she is trying to make. The way this woman's been treated in childbirth means that she is not fully aware of what actually happened to her, and she can't make any unbiased opinion, or decision, of her own. She's really having it made for her by the medical profession. The reason so many women feel differently may be because they've never had the chance either.

Chairman: Do you think that pain here is being used as a symbol of what the whole 'childbirth business' means to a woman?

Rod: No, I think the woman relating this experience has really got herself in a knot. She's saying that a woman should be able to feel pain so that she knows what she's going through, and so that she might make the decision not to do it again. But if a woman doesn't feel any pain directly, then she can equally make the decision about whether or not she wants to go ahead with it again.

Liz: But how do you know . . .

Tony: I think the implication is that she feels the pain while she is giving birth, then forgets it afterwards. The case is almost true of any pain which is relieved. I know I have experienced pain and afterwards you don't think about it again unless you get in the same situation. It's something you push into the back of your mind. It's not something you sit back and think about.

Robert: Certainly with the pain of childbirth a woman experiences incredible pain. But I have been told by quite a few women that they completely forget about the pain altogether and the joy of bearing the child completely overwhelms it.

Hilary: It would depend on their attitude to the child, wouldn't it?

Robert: Well, in most cases with most women I think that would be the case, wouldn't you?

Rod: Some women say there's not much pain involved anyway.

Chairman: Isn't that arguing against the point you were making before?

Rod: No; why should it affect a woman's choice that she hasn't felt the pain? Why should that affect a woman's choice about whether or not she wanted to have another baby or not? Why should a woman have to choose only after having experienced the pain of childbirth? Why can't she have a painless delivery and choose on that?

Liz: The point she is trying to make is that pain might be a deterrent to having babies. Whether that is true or false I don't know. I think it is false.

Nicholas: The answer to Rod's argument is in the passage. It is saying that the woman doesn't get any choice, because the system is such that she never experiences the pain and . . .

Liz: No; she experiences the pain but doesn't remember it, that's what it is saying.

Nicholas: But look, the passage says 'I thought it sounded just like the sort of drug a man would invent'. This is a strongly feminist argument. It's basically saying that men control the functions of women by never letting them have the choice.

Chairman: How would you answer that Rod?

Rod: I think this woman just has a hang-up about having children.

Hilary: Yeah, that's exactly the point!

Robert: This woman sounds like she has had a really terrible childbirth herself. She knows what she felt and is really frightened of it, and now says everyone else should have the right to be frightened of it as well.

Chairman: All right; the narrator is putting forward an opinion which some of us agree with, some of us disagree with, and some of us don't think is valid.

Tony: What about the last lines in the first paragraph: 'she really didn't know what she was doing because she was in a kind of twilight sleep'. It's more than pain. It was degrading that a woman should, at a time when she should be most aware and most alert to what is going on around her, be put in this sort of condition. She's treated like a little girl and told what to do. She is given orders. And it seems to me that this is part of the experience of having a child.

Robert: I agree.

David: Pain has its own anaesthetic sort of effect anyway. You lose your awareness of other things that are going on around you and you are not conscious in the normal way. You are not free to concentrate on anything else, so really you wouldn't necessarily be making a 'free' decision while experiencing pain.

Chairman: What about the last few lines in the passage: 'the drug would make her forget how bad the pain had been, when all the time, in some secret part of her, that long, blind, doorless and windowless corridor of pain was waiting to open up and shut her in again'. Now what does that mean? Is that metaphorical?

David: Yes, I think that's a very good metaphor, the endless corridor of pain.

Chairman: What could she be talking about?

Robert: Well, it could represent a patient's experience of being trolleyed down to theatre, or down a hospital corridor.

David: Or could it mean when you're having pain, it just seems to go on, and on, and you don't know when it's going to end—it's just an endless tunnel, there's no escape.

Chairman: Do you think she could be talking about her genital 'corridor'?

Gillian (smiling): Yes, she could.

The next passage discussed was from Charles Lamb's essay, 'The Convalescent'.

He has put on the strong armour of sickness, he is wrapped in the callous hide of suffering; he keeps his sympathy, like some curious vintage, under trusty lock and key, for his own use only.

He lies pitying himself, honing and moaning to himself; he yearneth over himself; his bowels are even melted within him, to think what he suffers; he is not ashamed to weep over himself.

He is forever plotting how to do some good to himself; studying little strategems and artificial alleviations . . .

To the world's business he is dead. He understands not what the callings and occupations of mortals are; only he has a glimmering conceit of some such thing, when the doctor makes his daily call: and even in the lines of that busy face he reads no multiplicity of patients, but solely conceives of himself as *the sick man.*[3]

Chairman: What does this passage mean?

Brendan: I think it is mainly about the self-focusing that goes on when you're ill. You stop communicating with the worldly things around you. I think this is a fairly common response for patients who are ill.

Rod: No; it would be about fifty-fifty.

Doug: It depends on the character of the patient.

Hilary: A lot of patients compare themselves to the patients in the next bed. They look at them and say, 'Well I thought I was sick until I saw them, and now I think perhaps I was being selfish.'

Brendan: Many people put on a cheerful exterior; they're bright, and, just as the passage says, they have on a strong armour of sickness. We, as doctors, can go around thinking that patient's O.K., he's smiling and sitting back and seems happy. But really he's crying out.

Liz: I was going to make a similar point to Brendan. Quite often I have sort of assumed that the patient was all right, and then they really shock you one day. You think a patient is coping all right, and then you get talking to them . . .

Robert: Yes, time and time again they break down while we are talking to them.

Chairman: Given that there's some truth in the feeling that patients who are sick do get more self-orientated, what is the practical importance of this for a doctor in the ward?

David: It means that you just can't stand there, you've got to reach out to a patient.

Brendan: Yes, and it means that you have to specifically ask the patients what *their* problems are. You've got to give them time. You can't rush them, you've got to give them time to say something if they want to say something.

Rod: And you've got to give them their privacy.

Brendan: Sometimes a patient sits there turning a lot of things over in their mind.

Chairman: That's a good phrase, 'turning things over in their mind'. What sort of things might a patient be worrying over which a doctor may not be aware of?

David: A sick patient might read things into every little nuance of a doctor's actions. The patient might believe that the doctor is thinking this or that and may misinterpret things which the doctor doesn't even notice he's doing. He may think the doctor believes he is going to die.

Tony: If a doctor goes in and spends two minutes with one patient and ten minutes with another, this can be misinterpreted.

Liz: I think that during a ward round, when the medical staff has been standing around a bed talking, and talking about something that that particular patient doesn't really have, the effect is fearful. Mentioning 'cancer' or a diagnosis which has nothing to do with that patient, is unkind.

Chairman: Are there any other things which go on routinely in a ward which a patient might be upset about or misinterpret?

Gillian: I would hate to be a boarder in a ward in which I didn't belong. Boarders get a raw deal. All they ever get told is that their own doctor will come around soon; the doctors who belong to that ward say, 'Oh, look, we're not sure about you, we don't know anything about you. You'll have to wait until your own doctor comes around.' They don't even fit into the ward. I'd hate to be a boarder.

Chairman: So we believe that self-orientation, at least to some extent, is a common part of the experience of being ill. But does this self-concern always need to be selfish?

Brendan: No, it's human.

Nicholas: Yes; a husband who's ill might be concerned about his wife or his family. He might be concerned about how his illness would affect them.

Chairman: Rod mentioned the importance of privacy in illness. Could we look at the next passage in relation to that. It comes from Virginia Woolf's essay, 'On Being Ill'.

> We do not know our own souls, let alone the souls of others. Human beings do not go hand in hand the whole stretch of the way. There is virgin forest in each; a snowfield where even the print of birds' feet is unknown. Here we go alone, and like it better so. Always to have sympathy, always to be accompanied, always to be understood would be intolerable. But in health the genial pretence must be kept up and the effort renewed—to communicate, to civilise, to share, to cultivate the desert, educate the native, to work together by day and by night to sport. In illness this make-believe ceases.[4]

Chairman: Stuart, would you like to start?

Stuart: I think there's one bit that I do like in this passage: 'always to be understood would be intolerable.' I think that's a good comment because there are so many times when nurses and doctors say, 'There, there, that's all right, it's O.K.' It's very condescending to a patient who doesn't really understand, and who sits there in silence. But for someone who *is* aware of what's going on, to have people around pandering to them, patting them on the back and giving them the superficial reassurance, I think it would be very upsetting.

Robert: Yes, there's a lot of cliches like 'things will be all right'.

Dave: One of the things that really drives me mad in films and in soppy movies is when somebody is dying and the mother-in-law comes along and says, [*exaggerated tone*] 'Oh, you'll be all right tomorrow', and you know that they're 'cactus'.

Chairman: 'Cactus?' What on earth does that mean?

Dave: That means they've had it.

Chairman: Oh, I see—the generation gap!

[*Laughter*]

Brendan: Coming back to the passage, I'm not sure that the 'make-believe' does cease.

Liz: For some people I think it does, but for other people, they do like to be alone.

Brendan: In other cases the make-believe takes off very strongly.

Chairman: Isn't that a separate point? There is a make-believe in relation to life in general which stops. There is another make-believe which starts in relation to a patient's denial of their illness. Is this second sort of make-believe the point Virginia Woolf is making?

Brendan: No, I agree. It's a different point.

David: One of the things with all of these extracts is that none of them would apply to all patients in all circumstances.

Chairman: Absolutely.

David: All of them seem to be from a personal viewpoint.

Chairman: And they're not all true in all cases.

David: Yes.

Chairman: I would hate to think that any of these passages were recommended as 'laws of human nature'. Each one of us will read them differently. There is individuality here in the passages. There's individuality in the fourteen or fifteen of us around this table, and there's individuality in everyone of the thirty-one patients in our wards. *That* is the point.

David: And isn't that part of what she is saying—that people are individuals?

Chairman: I think so.

Jane: I was just thinking that in relation to privacy in illness, the hospital environment usually prevents it. It's almost impossible, because in a hospital environment there are just so many people involved, all trying to help you. You don't really get a chance to think for yourself. You're woken up in the morning and washed and fed just when it is convenient for somebody else, not when you'd like to be.

Rod: But on the other hand, hospital can be a very lonely place. You can spend a lot of time by yourself. Just the fact that there are a lot of people there, who are only taking a superficial interest, doesn't mean companionship.

Chairman: Good. Well what is Virginia Woolf suggesting on that point when she says, 'in health the genial pretence must be kept up . . . In illness this make-believe ceases'?

Rod: I think what she's saying is that when you're healthy, if you want to go off and sit down by yourself and not talk to anyone, everyone looks at you and thinks that you're a bit queer; but when you're sick everyone expects you to go off and sit down by yourself and not talk to anyone.

Liz: I disagree with Rod's comment that in sickness you are 'expected' to go off and sit by yourself.

Chairman: Rod has given one interpretation. Could there be any others?

Stuart: I think you could look at this a different way. I think it is a comment on human relationships too, because she says the 'human beings do not go hand in hand the whole stretch of the way'. And . . .

Chairman: Is that true?

Stuart: Well, I am just commenting on what *she* said. She is saying that illness in itself is 'the virgin forest and the snowfield', and no one really knows how they are going to react to it. She says that a human relationship, or going hand in hand with someone else (superficially most of the time), is not sufficient to cover the bleak situation when you are ill, because you are by yourself. I think that's the significance of the passage—the sort of desolate scenes implied by 'the virgin forest'.

Chairman: Is 'a virgin forest', 'a snowfield where even the print of birds' feet is unknown', meant to signify a desolate thing?

Several students [*together*]: No . . . the snowfield doesn't mean sickness, it means the private territory in a person, — . . . it sounds like there's something sacred about it.

Nicholas: Isn't she saying that in a sickness you lose a lot of your rights? You lose the right to your inner self and more or less everything is done for you. Whereas in health that is not the case.

Rod: No; I think she's saying the opposite of that. She's saying that in health you've got to keep up the genial pretence of being social, but in illness this make-believe, this pretence, is gone—and you can be yourself.

Gillian: She's saying it's nasty in health; everyone's dishonest about everyday life, but in sickness that ends.

Chairman: Speaking as a group member, I would feel that Rod and Gillian are close to the meaning of the passage—that in health we have the resources and the energy to keep up the pretence in being social, but when we get sick an element of 'well I just can't be bothered now' creeps in.

Gillian: Yes, I agree with that.

Tony: It's very pessimistic. One could make a distinction between the individuality of a person, and their intelligibility–what outsiders understand them to be. We seem to be talking all the time about individuality as if it were a part of the whole person which is untrespassable. But I don't see that at all; I don't see individuality as some sort of enigma which nobody else can understand except you. I think a person can be an individual, and, at the same time, still be understood.

Liz: I don't think she is making them the same thing . . .

Tony: Yes, but we have been talking about individuality . . .

Liz: She's saying that . . .

Rod: Only a part . . .

Liz: She's saying that only a part of a person is felt, by them, to be private.

Gillian: I think she is saying there is a part of individuality which most people wish to keep to themselves. I don't think that excludes them from having a shared individuality.

Brendan: I agree, individuality could be divided into that part which is shared with others and a part which is private.

Chairman: So what some of you seem to be saying is that inasmuch as there is a private aspect to most individuals, the passage is meaningful.

Nicholas: Provided we *are* clear about its meaning! Isn't she saying that in health individuality, or the pretence towards individuality, is maintained. I read the lines 'Always to have sympathy, always to be accompanied, always to be understood would be intolerable', to refer to sickness. Whereas in health you're not given sympathy. She is saying that in health you are not accompanied all the time, but it's in illness that this happens. Your individuality is trampled upon in illness.

Rod: No, she's saying in illness you can't be bothered with company and you get some individuality back.

Chairman: O.K. Well it's obvious we can read this passage in a number of ways. Whether or not the author intended ambiguity is a different thing. Ambiguity in writing can be intentional. Ambiguity, to some extent, is inherent in the use of metaphor, or in the sort of playing on words which Shakespeare did so well. Such ambiguity doesn't mean confusion. But if ambiguity becomes a barrier to understanding the meaning of a work, then it can be a criticism; and if there is any passage that we study which you feel to be so ambiguous as to be confusing, obviously that is a criticism of the writing.

From your comments you suggest that there could be multiple meanings in this particular passage. If that is so, then those of us who disagree have no right to hobnail our own opinion over somebody else's.

Nicholas: All I'd say is that my interpretation is a point for discussion, it seems a valid view to say that individuality is destroyed in hospital, which I think it is.

Rod: The argument against your interpretation, Nick, is to look at what the passage says, because it says '*In health* the genial pretence must be kept up and the effort renewed–to communicate, to civilise, to share,' and so on. Nick's interpretation is that in health the genial pretence of individuality is what is being kept up. But it is not, it's the genial pretence to communicate, and to civilize, and to share. That's what she is saying, it's there!

Nicholas: Well, I'm sorry. I was more interested in the overall argument than the trimmings.

Chairman: Does anyone else want to make a comment on this passage now?

Students: No.

Chairman: One of the loose objectives of this course is to introduce you to the idea that in thinking about human issues, science is deficient. There is no way that Rod could prove to Nicholas that his 'feeling' for the passage is wrong, because his interpretation of the passage is partly personal. [*General laughter.*] For example, this sort of discussion is different from an argument about the dose of digitalis which you need to digitalize a patient. On that score, one person could prove to another person that the idea he had of the dose was wrong according to experiment and observation. On matters scientific, proof *is* the warrant of truth. On human issues however, we have the individuality of different opinions, different interpretations, and different sentiments. We anticipate and we alter. It's in this area that shades of meaning creep in. We will find that on many points both in these sessions and in our dealings with the views of our patients, we have to agree to disagree. We'll say, 'Well I just see it differently, but perhaps I'll think about it and tomorrow I'll feel more the truth of what someone else was saying.'

Robert: Yes, we'll both change our opinions and then we'll clash again.

[*General laughter.*]

Chairman: Just a moment ago Rod made a point on the solitude which can be experienced during illness. This leads us into the next passage which makes a delicate point on one effect of the solitude offered by illness. The passage is from André Gide's novel *The Immoralist*.

There is nothing more tragic for a man who has been expecting to die than a long convalescence. After that touch from the wing of Death, what seemed important is so no longer; other things become so which had at first seemed unimportant, or which one did not even know existed. The miscellaneous mass of acquired knowledge of every kind that has overlain the mind gets peeled off in places like a mask of paint, exposing the bare skin—the very flesh of the authentic creature that had lain hidden beneath it.

He it was whom I thenceforward set out to discover—that authentic creature, 'the old Adam'. . . . whom everything about me—books, masters, parents, and I, myself had begun by attempting to suppress. And he was already coming into view, still in the rough and difficult of discovery, thanks to all that overlay him, but so much the more worthy to be discovered, so much the more valorous. Thenceforward I despised the secondary creature, the creature who was due to teaching, whom education had painted on the surface. These overlays had to be shaken off.

And I compared myself to a palimpsest; I tasted the scholar's joy when he discovers under more recent writing, and on the same paper, a very ancient and infinitely more precious text.[5]

Chairman: Who can give us a paraphrase of the human experience being related in this passage?

Tony: A man who is confronting death realizes that his previous conduct, his thoughts and so on, have been pointless, and have been worthless to him. Now he's trying to discover something worthwhile in himself—what is called the authentic creature.

Chairman: Good. And what sort of feelings does the experience being related create in you?

[*Long pause.*]

David: It seems like necessity. It is something that he seems to find traumatic, but necessary.

Robert: It's almost a revolution.

Colin: He's more or less in a new environment and he needs new tools to handle it. He seems to be searching for these. His new environment is that he faced death, and the things which he has used to adapt and cope with life are no help because he is in a different context now. He has to cope with dying.

Brendan: He's not dying, he's facing a long convalescence.

Colin: Yes, yes, he's facing a long convalescence. That's what I meant.

Nicholas: I get a spiritual sense from this passage, almost something holy going on. He's talking really about a reincarnation. It's the same body but it's now got a different view.

Gillian: I don't think it's a *different* view because he now has become really what he always was. It's just that everything that was on the surface and meaningless has gone. I don't think it's a reincarnation insofar as it's not a new person. He's showing that he has become what he has been all along.

Chairman: All this has happened during an episode of illness: the self-questioning, the reorientation. The 'essential Adam' or the 'original him' is now standing up to be counted. I don't believe that this is a very common occurrence in medical practice, but when it occurs it can be one of the most profound experiences in the life of the human being concerned. Such a man or a woman could go back in to society quite a different individual. During such an episode, a patient can make decisions in relation to their work, their family, their friends, or their sense of self. Their values can change. I am offering an opinion. Does anyone disagree with it?

David: I agree. It's just like Scrooge after the three hauntings in Dickens' *The Christmas Carol*. And I remember seeing an interview with a heart-transplant patient where he seemed to be saying exactly what you have said. He said, 'When I mow the lawn now, I notice the smell of it, and when I do things I notice more what I am doing. I notice there are clouds in the sky and things moving. I didn't have this sort of view before.'

Stuart: There are two attitudes which can be taken when facing death. One is to accept it philosophically; the other is the materialistic attitude of someone who now has a set limit on how long they are going to live, and who takes the opportunity to do everything that they have always wanted to do, but never could because they didn't have the money. Now their life is going to end, they can spend what they've got.

Chairman: Does the group feel this happens? Commonly?

Male student: Yes, I think it's a lot more common than what the passage is saying.

Gillian: Oh I don't. I think most people keep going with what they are doing—they don't want to be reminded of their illness.

Brendan: I agree with Gillian. Patients don't want to have it put in their mind all the time that they are going to die.

Chairman: How would you answer that Stuart?

Stuart: I don't know! It's another point of view, I suppose every patient is a different case.

Chairman: All right, well what sort of patients could be particularly liable to undergo the experience that Gide has related?

Rod: A patient with a heart attack, or a perforated ulcer. Where a way of life has contributed to the actual illness.

Tony: An acute alcoholic with, say, an acute attack of hepatitis or pancreatitis.

Chairman: Or perhaps a patient who has become trapped by the way he has been living. And might there be any liabilities from this particular experience?
Stuart: He might go through all the problems of finding his real self and then die.

[*General laughter.*]

Brendan: It might affect his family.
Liz: Yes, he might reject what he had before and finish up with nothing.
Tony: He might become vulnerable to a whole lot of suspect religious codes.
Chairman: You say vulnerable, are you making a judgement on these religious codes?
Tony: Yes, it's me passing a judgement of those particular sects.
Chairman: Well do we have the right to make that sort of judgement on the followers of, say, Hare Krishna for example? We might think them strange, but on the other hand they would say they are happy!
Tony: Perhaps not so much Hare Krishna but there are some other sinister sects.
Jane: A patient's previous way of life may have been very adaptive: he's been living in society a certain way, and now he's changing his ideas. He could have a lot of difficulty fitting back into the society he knew.
Chairman: Does the group feel that there is a fundamental conflict between an individual's sense of self and the demands society makes on him?

[*General agreement.*] Yes; absolutely.

Chairman: Does anyone know, in this particular passage, what this man's self-finding involved?
Tony: Was he a homosexual?
Chairman: Yes, that was the situation in this extract. For other patients the experience could mean finding themselves vocationally, finding themselves in terms of their family, their creativity, their recreational activities, or their spirit and soul.

Now, as I said before, I'm not saying that the particular experience we are discussing is common in illness, but it does happen. And so I feel that if this particular aspect of the experience of being ill hasn't been covered anywhere else in your course, then we were right to consider it now. Very occasionally a patient might say to you during the course of their illness, 'I've been thinking about the way I've been living.' Behind that comment may be something as profound as what we have been discussing here.

There are many situations in life besides sickness which can bring about self-questioning: isolation, change of location, any sort of setback or grief, and 'crisis' periods of life. Convalescence offers the opportunity of time to reflect, and privacy.

Male student: Not always.

Chairman: I agree, not always. Are there any aspects of hospital life where this is not so?

Gillian: Outpatients.

Chairman: Go on.

Gillian: It's so degrading! There is very little privacy, everyone can hear what is being said, and half the time you are exposed in the cubicles while you are being examined.

Tony: I think patients are being kept waiting too long there. They sit around in the corridor in great numbers, sometimes their history is lost, or people say, 'You shouldn't be here', or 'You're in the wrong clinic', and the whole experience is just unpleasant. Dehumanizing.

Gillian: I think it's dishonest too, because when students examine the patient they really aren't doing anything. The patient doesn't know that they're students, and you feel like you are deceiving them when you sit down and talk to them. They've come with a worry and they think you are going to do something about it and you are really only using them as a learning object.

Liz: Yes, it seems to me that very little is done in Outpatients. It's just like a sorting ground.

Brendan: I agree, it's dehumanizing.

Hilary: I think most patients in Outpatients, or many patients in Outpatients, feel that they are not being listened to, they have worries and concerns which are missed by the doctor. The doctor is sometimes preoccupied with the medical aspects and the patient's own little concern is just passed over.

Chairman: That's something we are going to discuss in Session 5, Hilary. It's a good point.

All right, now let's move on to something a little more modern and consider a passage from *Brian's Wife, Jenny's Mum*, a group of essays and poems written by suburban women.

> The money's good when you work full time. Mind you, you get bloody tired, working full time. It would be nice if you could just sit down to a meal when you get home instead of having to get it ready first. Then you could gather your resources together to enable you to get on after tea with the housework, the washing, the ironing that you didn't do during the day, even, hopefully, prepare tomorrow night's meal –a casserole, a curry, a pie, a stew, so that all you will have to do is heat it up when you come home, peel some potatoes and put them on, whip up an easy dessert. But most of the women

I know, who work full time, say they don't bother with dessert any more. Buy a bit of cake on the way home. Oh, they never *make* cake any more. They've got more to do with their time than bake a cake. Five minutes after you've taken it out of the oven it's gone. At least when you buy it, it lasts longer. Oh, they eat eventually. They'll eat anything if they're hungry enough. Although when they get that hungry they usually go down the street and buy some fish and chips. They make you wonder whether cooking a meal is worth it. It's handy to have a fish and chip shop nearby. . . .

I wouldn't be without my tablets, either, but they're not the same thing [as next-door's]. She takes hers all day long. I have one in the morning when I get up, one at teatime and one when I go to bed. I might need one at lunchtime. But they keep me going.

Of course, I know I'm not really going anywhere. I mean, where is anybody going? You are born, you grow up, you get married, you have kids and they grow up and get married and have kids. You die. There's not much to it really, is there? Just days. Days to get through. Christmas to Christmas. Birthday to Birthday. But you try to forget about those. You get a nice present, a card from your husband, from the kids. But you're always another year older. You know where you're going all right. Suburban neurosis?

Yes, I suppose that's what it's about. Just life.[6]

[*During the reading of this passage there were numerous chuckles of genuine laughter from the students.*]

Chairman: O.K. girls, do you want to start?

Robert: Are these different sections from the same passage?

Chairman: Yes, they are all paragraphs from the same passage.

David: I think that third paragraph is fairly amazing. I mean if I stop and think sometimes I get into that sort of circle. [*General laughter.*] You're born, you get married, you grow up, you have kids, and they grow up and get married and have kids, and they die and there is not much more to it . . .

Liz: There's tremendous disillusionment in this passage.

Chairman: Is this a common problem, this 'suffering of being'?

David: Yes, very!

Chairman: And what's the medical significance of this?

David: The depressed housewife needing Valium, and Bex, and aspirin.

Dave [*speaking theatrically*]: Oh these aren't Bex, these are 'something different to next-door's'.

Chairman: And, what's the medical answer to this problem?

Tony: Well, it's a difficult situation, but—perhaps to help a woman like this to communicate with other housewives, to do some courses.

[*General comment.*]

David [*raising his voice above the other voices*]: She's either bored, or she's unfulfilled, or both!
Stuart: There's nothing a bullet wouldn't fix!
Chairman: A what?
Stuart: A bullet.

[*Raucous laughter.*]

Chairman: Fired by the doctor, by her, or by you? Are you implying a serious point Stuart?

[*General laughter.*]

Stuart: Well, it would certainly put a stop to the continuous circle! It would produce a premature end really!

[*Pause in the discussion.*]

Liz: I don't think there's much you can do in a situation like this. It's important to have companionship in a situation like this, to have somebody else to talk to and communicate with, but as far as fixing up their whole life, that's difficult.
Chairman: A woman can get pretty tired of communicating with a three-year-old!
Stuart: And a three-year-old probably gets bored too.
Nicholas: In more than just a straight medical sense, one approach that has been widely used is the Women's Health Centre approach. It started in many areas where you have a collective of people who have very certain ideas on how society should operate. The object is re-education, and when women come with problems to these places, educative help is offered.
Stuart: There's also a cultural problem here. Although this woman thinks she's in a rut, there are a great number of European women, Italians or Greeks, and so on, who would accept this as normal. They would accept it whole-heartedly and would be totally out of place doing anything else. You would probably cause just as much anxiety and neurosis if you tried to put them in any other sort of context.
Liz: The weirdness of all of this is that when you're depressed you see this vicious circle, and then, what amazes me, is that when you're not depressed, you're quite happy to lead exactly the same life and it feels good to be alive. So if you can get over a patient's depression, that's what you should be combating, not trying to change their lives.
Tony: But don't you think the depression is inherent in the lifestyle?

Liz: Hmmm.
Stuart: No! Because a lot of people might . . .
Chairman: Might it become so?
Rod: If you tell people they are going to become depressed, they will become depressed.
Nicholas [*firmly*]: Exactly! And the survival of this sort of horror depends on ignorance. I mean, if you're ignorant of the fact that you've got a lung cancer, you could be happy with that?
Rod, Liz, Robert, and Nicholas [*all trying to talk together*].
Chairman: Hilary, I see you trying to say something.
Hilary: If they are already dissatisfied, you can't make them satisfied no matter what you do or say to them.
Liz: But I'm suggesting that it's—yeah—all right.
David, Liz, and Rod [*all trying to talk together*].
Chairman: What would you say to a housewife who was sitting here saying, 'It's all very well for you to be discussing this nicely in the abstract, you just haven't experienced what we go through. You haven't experienced this draining way of life. You haven't experienced the degradation, the wanting to get out from this, but unable to because of society's expectations, or my commitment to the family. I've got three kids under five and my husband refuses to look after them to let me get out a bit.'
Robert: Yes, I think it is just part of the whole sick society's set-up.
Tony: The husband *is* the problem frequently, because he won't take any responsibility.
Rod: I disagree. I think it is just as bad for husbands . . . [*General laughter.*] The husbands have the same problem as the women. They have to go out to work, they get tired . . .
Gillian and Liz [*interjecting*]: . . . Yeah, they come home tired, but their dinner is ready and the house has been tidied.
David: Just a minute, this woman *is* going to work!
Many students [*trying to talk together*].
Rod: Yes, the husband has to come home and mow the lawn and wash the car and so on.
Liz: That's not what we are discussing at the moment, we are discussing the common situation that Dr Moore just outlined.
Rod: But this woman is talking as if it is only the poor female [*Male voice:* Yeah, that's right!] who's in a rut and has nothing to look forward to. But the hubby has the same lifestyle.
Liz [*interjecting*]: But I think that is irrelevant. We are discussing . . .
Rod [*continuing, flustered*]: The husband has the same sort of lifestyle—he goes down to the tote and puts on a bet, and then goes to the pub, goes home, goes to bed, gets up the next morning, goes to work, goes down to the tote—it's bad all round!
Liz [*trying unsuccessfully to speak*].

David: It's just that suburban marriage is mutually stifling to everybody. If you find that sort of thing stifling [*laughter*]. Some people get drunk and beat up their wife every night and some people enjoy it.

Chairman: Jane, I see you are wanting to say something.

Jane [*slowly*]: Hmm, no, I'm just listening.

Liz: The males here seem to be saying it doesn't matter if a woman's mind doesn't grow because of a lack of nutrition, but that it matters if the kids starve to death.

David: No, it doesn't matter about the kids because they are only going to grow up and have more kids and so on.

Liz: And they're going to be the same!

Chairman: Well, irrespective of our prejudices . . .

Liz: [*interrupting*]: But those prejudices are absolutely relevant.

Chairman [*continuing*]: Yes they are, absolutely relevant. But aside from those prejudices, this passage confronts us with a medical situation because doctors are prescribing drugs for just the sort of experience this woman is relating.

Now, time is so short, so let us close the session with a reading of a passage from one hundred years earlier. It reinforces the view that a certain way of living can be undermining, and yet the doctor may be called upon to support that way of life by prescribing drugs which allow people to cope with it. It also portrays that appalling state where a human being is without hope. It comes from Mrs Gaskell's novel *Mary Barton*, and concerns a man called John Barton, Mary's father. The novel was written in 1848.

> Then came a long period of bodily privation; of daily hunger after food; and though he tried to persuade himself he could bear want himself with stoical indifference, and did care about it as little as most men, yet the body took its revenge for its uneasy feelings. The mind became soured and morose, and lost much of its equipoise. It was no longer elastic, as in the days of youth, or in times of comparative happiness; it ceased to hope. And it is hard to live on when we can no longer hope.
>
> The same state of feeling which John Barton entertained, if belonging to one who had leisure to think of such things and physicians to give names to them, would have been called monomania; so haunting, so incessant, were the thoughts that pressed upon him. . . .
>
> It is true, much of their morbid power might be ascribed to the use of opium. But before you blame too harshly this use, or rather abuse, try a hopeless life, with daily cravings of the body for food. Try, not alone being without hope yourself, but seeing all around you reduced to the same despair, arising from the same circumstances; all around you telling (though they use no words or

> language), by their looks and feeble actions, that they are suffering and sinking under the pressure of want. Would you not be glad to forget life, and its burdens? And opium gives forgetfulness for a time.[7]

Chairman: Now, I'll just leave that passage with you to think about, and to see if you feel there is a modern equivalent, or modern significance of the message contained in it.

Nicholas: One point in relation to that passage is an argument brought up by Illich in his book *Medical Nemesis.* His argument is that the industrial society causes a lot of the illness, and all that doctors do is prescribe and legitimize illness. They don't try to change the society which is causing all the distress.

Rod: Is it our job to change society?

Nicholas [*continuing*]: We are busily engaged in just propping up the situation.

Chairman: Could I comment on Rod's point about whether it's a doctor's job to change society. In Session 6 we shall be coming back to a consideration of the relationship between society and medicine through some passages in Chekhov's short stories. So perhaps we can hold that discussion till then.

Well, I think we are all getting pretty tired now so let's call it a day for this session.

ESSAY 1

THE SIGNIFICANCE OF SUFFERING

The same nerves are fashioned to sustain
The greatest pleasure and the greatest pain.[1]
Samuel Garth

As young doctors and nurses it takes us many years to learn that each patient we care for has very personal and private feelings during his or her illness. Patients are extremely alert to any aspect of the doctor's conversation or the nurses' concern which affects them, and have a great awareness of every indelicacy which takes place at their bedside. A patient's mind can magnify beyond belief little acts to which the busy doctor gives only passing consideration: 'Why is my bed being moved to that corner?'; 'What on earth is a *toilet* operation?'; 'Why am I the last case on the operating list?'; 'Why did the doctor attend to that patient before me?'; 'What do they mean by a special test?'; 'Why did he ask if anybody in the family has had it?'; 'Why did he ask about my children?'; 'Why did he have a piteous look on his face when he asked me do I have any relatives?'; 'How can he say "Don't be worried" when he looked worried?'; 'Why does he want to see me again if everything really is all right?'

Separated from everyday distractions and looking quietly at a colourless hospital wall, a patient finds his thoughts dwell and delve, plunging down paths of self-concern which the busy doctor, who has others on his mind, often overlooks. One of the rewards to be gained from our attempt at human understanding is that we can frequently appreciate some of our patients' thoughts and fears. We can perceive what it means to have one's vigour and youth subverted by sickness or to have one's mature aspirations undermined by disease. We can appreciate the pain of having one's closest and most special relationship torn apart by the threat of death, or to have the person closest to us—the one with whom we share our life's purpose—left alone when we are destroyed by some awful erosion.

In their early days at the hospital, young medical students and doctors have some difficulty in understanding the thoughts and fears of elderly patients: their concern about an afterlife, their feelings of guilt and shame, and their need to have things explained gently.

Clinical events should always proceed slowly for it is bad medical practice to spring things on aged patients. They should always be allowed the time to get used to the idea of any procedure or programme which the doctor has in mind for them. But the major medical demand of caring for old people is to have the perception and insight necessary to appreciate their fears of loneliness, of dependency, and of uselessness. Something which is often underestimated is the very touching love that can exist between very elderly partners who have lived to an age where the doubts and disillusionments of life have left their scars. I believe that the younger the doctor is, the more difficulty he has in appreciating the special problems of being old.

We ask a great deal of our young doctors. We ask them to cope with a science which eludes even the experienced, and human experiences which elude all.

Young patients are another special group. They frequently feel that disease is both a spoiler and a restraint for it reduces their personal freedom to work, to engage, to create, and to romp. The young are frequently bewildered and uncommunicative during their illness; they are agitated, and restless to escape from the thraldom of infirmity. They fear physical mutilation.

The experience of illness can produce a sense of remoteness from the familiar and closeness to the rare. The advent of television in hospital wards has removed much of the feeling of dislocation from time which can take place in hospitals. Patients who watch television have their evenings timetabled to the same pattern as in health. They are spared that sense of separation from the events of the outside world. And they frequently laugh. But not all patients avoid that strange sense of alienation produced by hospitalization, and this is particularly so for long-term patients. In his Nobel Prize-winning novel *The Magic Mountain*, Thomas Mann portrays this experience.

> For the moment we need only recall the swift flight of time–even of a quite considerable period of time–which we spend in bed when we are ill. All days are nothing but the same day repeating itself–or rather, since it is always the same day, it is incorrect to speak of repetition; a continuous present, and identity, an everlastingness–such words as these would better convey the idea . . .
>
> Vacuity, monotony, have, indeed, the property of lingering out the moment and the hour and of making them tiresome. But they are capable of contracting and dissipating the larger, the very large time-units, to the point of reducing them to nothing at all. And conversely, a full and interesting content can put wings to the hour of the day; yet it will lend to the general passage of time a weightiness, a breadth and solidity which cause even the eventful years to flow far more slowly than those poor, bare, empty ones over which the wind passes and they are gone . . .

> Habituation is a falling asleep or fatiguing of the sense of time; which explains why young years pass slowly, while later life flings itself faster and faster upon its course. We are aware that the intercalation of periods of change and novelty is the only means by which we can refresh our sense of time, strengthen, retard, and rejuvenate it, and therewith renew our perception of life itself. Such is the purpose of our changes of air and scene, of all our sojourns at cures and bathing resorts; it is the secret of the healing power of change and incident.[2]

So much of medical practice that we experience outside the great hospitals has an element of this disease, *life tiredness*, in its cause. So many of the everyday problems of people stem from the appalling boredom and sameness of their lives. As busy doctors and nurses engaged in stimulating work—without a moment available for commonplace boredom—it is not always easy for us to experience the *ennui* of life. Yet so many of our patients are failing through sheer fatigue. They experience the 'suffering of being' every day, without prospect or promise of release. For them, time is a tyranny, a master whose hands strike at their lives with incessantly cruel chimes. For them, life is a wound spring, a mortal coil, which twists the spirit from their souls. They are degraded by their own sense of useless monotony. They have little hope.

During our first discussion on the experience of illness we considered the fear, the isolation, and the degradation which can be part of that experience. I shall not reconsider those problems in this short essay. Instead I would like to explore some relatively neglected aspects of illness.

Medical men and women are practical people. The end point of their vocational energy is immediate, applied, and dominated by the consequences of their actions. This is part of the contract of therapeutic trust. This concept of consequence is sown into the furrows of the medical mind, so that doctors feel uneasy when straying into those pastures which put aside immediate effect and practical consequence, and instead germinate long-term reflection and theoretical speculation.

In our profession tacit assent is given to the exclusive view that disease degrades human beings, that it is bad, and that it should be corrected or eliminated wherever detected. To hold this view exclusively is to confess philosophical naïveté and simplicity. It is to adhere to an opinion that is unworthy of the reality.

I would agree that the commonest view of illness is that it is a malevolent force. Most people in our society do not view illness as something refined or worthy of reverence, but rather as a degrader of mankind—a degrader which is painful and offensive. Most patients who have an ongoing illness feel that their affliction has taken hold of them and has stained them. They feel spoiled. All human beings are slaves to hope and fear, and most concede that in the arithmetic of illness, one adds and multiplies human woes, one does not subtract or divide.

Now I am not saying that disease does not degrade and spoil human bodies, or that it does not reduce human pleasures and aspirations, or that it does not confine human capacity and freedom—it can and does most horribly. Nor am I saying that the health profession should not aim to alleviate such afflictions. What I am saying is that the experience of illness can do much more. It is these neglected or ignored aspects that I wish to highlight.

One admits an extreme lack of sensitivity and perception if, as a doctor, one fails to receive the full compass of experience that can take an ill patient beyond simple feelings of degradation or restriction. The experiences of illness are protean. In some cases disease can dignify, in others it creates heroic capacities. It can lead to self-realization; it can level unequal men; it can be thought of as an agent of retribution. It can be viewed as a helpful symptom in the identification of a deep social disorder, or even as an irritation which interferes with social productivity and prosperity. In other words it has many additional personal and social dimensions.

Even patients who see disease as a despoiler often experience sentiments of greater complexity. They see illness as an ever-present reminder of the unexpected, and of man's fundamental vulnerability. 'The actual tragedies of life bear no relation to one's preconceived ideas. In the event one is always bewildered by their simplicity, their grandeur of design, and by the element of the bizarre which seems inherent in them.'[3] Seneca, the Roman stoic philosopher, knew something of this experience:

> What is quite unlooked for is more crushing in its effect, and unexpectedness adds to the weight of disaster . . . We should project our thoughts ahead of us at every turn and have in mind every possible eventuality instead of the usual course of events . . . Misfortune has a way of choosing some unprecendented means or other of impressing its power on those who might have forgotten it. A single day strews in ruins all that was raised by a train of construction extending over a long span of time.[4]

A single motor accident, one hospital laboratory test, an emergency operation, each can raze to ruin all that was raised by the total of a man's life.

Illness frequently stimulates a busy man or woman to pause and reflect on the transience of life and the smallness of personal achievements, for, 'all the works of mortal man lie under the sentence of mortality; we live among things that are destined to perish'.[5] If a doctor or nurse takes the time, it is remarkable how many patients, in a quiet moment, will confess that they see their illness as a reminder of their own vulnerability in the face of larger than human forces. The Christian sentiment of divine retribution is often felt even by secular patients who see their illness as a punishment for some secret transgression. Disease is then the judiciary, passing the sentence and condemning the patient to some cell. Guilt and shame are added to the experience of being ill.

Another experience which can partner an episode of illness is a personal confrontation with the meaning and purpose of the life the patient has been living. I believe this is something which doctors and nurses learn with difficulty. An episode of illness frequently separates a person from his supporting environment. When that is gone, he loses a prop which acted as a defence against certain personal challenges and questions which—until that moment—had been pushed aside as too painful or too threatening. Stripped of the support of everyday hustle and business, a patient frequently finds that questions or confrontations which have been shirked rear up and demand recognition. Sometimes a patient *has* the courage to confront his whole identity—his beliefs, his standards, his aspirations and ambitions—but more commonly he is too vulnerable to undertake such a task.

The excursion in the patient's mind which creates such a questioning is mysterious. Listen to how Tolstoy describes the event for the ailing Prince in *War and Peace*:

> His mind was not in a normal state. A healthy man usually thinks of, feels, and remembers, innumerable things simultaneously, but has the power and will to select one sequence of thoughts or events on which to fix his whole attention. A healthy man can tear himself away from the deepest reflections to say a civil word to someone who comes in, and can then return again to his own thoughts. But Prince Andrew's mind was not in a normal state in that respect. All the powers of his mind were more active and clearer than ever, but they acted apart from his will. Most diverse thoughts and images occupied him simultaneously. At times his brain suddenly began to work with a vigour, clearness, and depth it had never reached when he was in health, but suddenly in the midst of its work it would turn to some unexpected idea and he had not the strength to turn it back again.[6]

I believe that such personal explorations are some of the most valuable, and, at the same time, disturbing moments in a person's life, for they can result in a considerable sense of conflict and challenge. That they occur during episodes of illness has been recorded in many diaries and autobiographies, and in many works of literature. In clinical practice they can be shared by any gentle and perceptive doctor or nurse who takes a moment to sit and talk with a patient who seems a little quieter than usual, whose book rests open and unturned while he gazes beyond the window, or who expresses a thought or asks a question which is felt to be out of character. It is difficult for a patient to communicate the experience of the reappraisal of his life which has been caused by an episode of illness. The words do not exist to express such a personal revolution or renaissance. Medical people should not intrude into this territory of personal experience unless invited. In our first session we considered the self-revelation and redirection which can occur during sickness. It was the sentiment captured so brilliantly in the passage from Andre Gide's novel, *The Immoralist*. Such an event may result in a reallocation of human and emotional priorities. Someone who was alienated from a patient may be reclaimed into his affections, and someone endeared may be rejected.

Disease can occasionally promote a spirit of togetherness in those who are like afflicted. The whole family of clubs and societies which bond together people with similar health liabilities is witness to this sentiment. Colostomy associations, ileostomy associations, clubs for amputees, groups trying to counteract the problems of obesity, alcoholism, and drug addiction are as important as any purely 'medical' contribution to the management of the patient's problems.

Illness or adversity can sometimes stimulate a social dimension of togetherness. Societies under the threat of a plague or pestilence share a common fear, and are frequently thrown together in a spirit of corporate unity against that common threat. Occasionally, as portrayed in Camus's book *The Plague*, it causes the disintegration of a society.

Let us consider a new thought. That part of the Christian belief which claims that there is virtue in self-denial and suffering has, in past ages, elevated physical affliction to a symbol of righteousness. It was seen as a burden to be borne, a gesture of the power of a demanding God. The spiritual dimension of a man enabled him to evade the physical consequences of suffering through a negation of his body (both Socrates and Christ were examples and, although somewhat exceptional, were not unique). For the spiritual or philosophical man is outside his body and beyond the immediacies of illness. As Thomas Mann wrote: 'A human being who is first of all an invalid is *all* body; therein lies his inhumanity and his debasement. In most cases he is little better than a carcass.'[7]

I know that formal religion is out of fashion in the Western world, and that man's religiosity is lying dormant. I also know that a modern man who undertakes a philosophical or spiritual exploration is regarded as 'suspect'. But the truth remains that, insofar as we are materialists, insofar as we are worldly and man orientated, insofar as we see the physicality of our bodies as our elemental part, then, so too, we shall suffer our illnesses without the assistance of our spiritual or philosophical capacity.

I have little liking for that aspect of the Christian tradition which elevates self-denial and self-restraint to the choicest expression of the human spirit. That is too negative for many modern people who would rather worship at the altar of self-fulfilment. Besides, it is inconsistent for a 'spiritual' man to elevate any aspect of the 'body'—even suffering. We have all experienced those patients who seem to have a philosophical attitude towards their disease. Some of them are religious, but many seem to draw on their own resources. Such patients, who are usually easy to look after, frequently win our admiration and respect. They also do a great deal to fortify the patients around them. On the other hand, patients who dwell excessively on their hardships, or who show little resolve in the face of their sickness, make mighty demands on our capacities of doctorship, and frequently irritate us.

Illness is a special time in the life of our patients. But it also produces disruptions, trials and anxieties in the relatives of those who are suffering. The next session with the students will consider the experience of illness from the relatives' point of view.

SESSION 2

THE RELATIVES' EXPERIENCE OF ILLNESS

Chairman: Today's topic is a consideration of the experience of illness from the relatives' point of view. This is an interesting topic from my point of view because you are the first group which has dealt with it. I haven't considered the extracts before, other than when I selected them, so we are all in the same boat today. I've added this particular topic because some students complained that they go through the whole of their medical course and the question of 'the relatives' just never comes up.

Let us start with a short extract. It comes from a story by Theodore Dreiser, 'The Lost Phoebe'.

> Old Henry Reifsneider and his wife Phoebe were a loving couple. You perhaps know how it is with simple natures that fasten themselves like lichens on the stones of circumstance and weather their days to a crumbling conclusion. The great world sounds widely, but it has no call for them. They have no soaring intellect. The orchard, the meadow, the cornfield, the pig-pen, and the chicken-lot measure the range of their human activities. When the wheat is headed it is reaped and threshed; when the corn is browned and frosted it is cut and shocked; when the timothy is in full head it is cut, and the haycock erected. After that comes winter, with the hauling of grain to market, the sawing and splitting of the wood, the simple chores of fire-building, meal-getting, occasional repairing, and visiting. Beyond these and the changes of weather–the snows, the rains, and the fair days–there are no immediate, significant things. All the rest of life is a far-off, clamorous phantasmagoria, flickering like Northern lights in the night, and sounding as faintly as cow-bells tinkling in the distance.
>
> Old Henry, who knew his wife would never leave him in any circumstances, used to speculate at times as to what he would do if she were to die. That was the one leaving that he really feared. As he climbed on the chair at night to wind the old, long-pendulumed, double-weighted clock, or went finally to the front and back door to

see that they were safely shut in, it was a comfort to know that Phoebe was there, properly ensconced on her side of the bed, and that if he stirred restlessly in the night, she would be there to ask what he wanted.[1]

Chairman: Who would like to start?

Dave: This is basically an extract about an old man and his wife who seem to be completely alienated from the rest of the world. They live in their own world and carry out their own simple chores. As far as they are concerned, the rest of the world is completely another thing. That seems to be the first paragraph. The second paragraph deals with the security he feels with his wife, and the sort of thoughts he would feel if she should die. That's a summary of the passage.

Chairman: What do you feel about the passage Dave?

Dave: I think it's quite moving. It's obvious that he is very attached to his wife. He needs her security, and as an outside observer I can see that one day he's going to be completely shattered when she dies.

Colin: I don't feel that it's all that moving. I think it's a very common experience, but there is an element of selfishness in it. Old Henry wants feed for his security, he's not concerned with what happens to her if he should die.

David: Yes, it's significant that it doesn't mention what happens if he should die first.

Chairman: The point you finished on Colin, the point of selfishness, is this characteristic of old people?

Colin: I think it's a natural response when two people who have been living together as long as one would imagine these two have. All they've really got is themselves. They have nothing else that they can hang on to.

Brendan: It's hardly selfishness to the exclusion of other things just because they are dependent on each other. They seem to be the sort of people, who, if a stranger turned up to their farm, would treat them hospitably and put them up.

Tony: It's sad that they have made such an investment in each other. It seems that if one were to leave or lose the other, then the surviving partner wouldn't be able to cope. I think it's a bad idea that people form such a close relationship.

Brendan [*together with many students*]: I disagree with that entirely.

Chairman: Tony, do you really believe that?

Tony: Yes, to some extent I do. I think there is a tendency towards isolation for couples who just live for themselves. I don't think it's morally wrong or anything like that. It just seems sad to me.

Chairman: Is this a paradox of human relationships: the greater the degree of commitment between two individuals, then the greater is the degree of vulnerability produced by the loss of a partner?

Tony: Yes it is. But what I am saying is that this sort of commitment carried too far can be dangerous.

Chairman: You seem to be suggesting that human relationships of this sort can be controlled; that an individual's power of reason can dictate the degree of their human and emotional involvement.

Tony: Well it can do, yes!

Hilary: I think this sort of relationship can become a vicious cycle in which they carry their dependence on each other too far. They seem to have so little else to depend upon and to preoccupy themselves with.

Chairman: Why do you think they have so little else?

Robert: One thing is they're isolated geographically living on a farm.

Chairman: Yes, this isolation might be as much a cause as an effect: the fact that they are separated from people would force them together more.

Colin: It also mentions that they have no soaring intellect. Simple people tend to be more dependent on each other.

Rod: I disagree with everyone when they suggest that this couple is isolated. They seem to be typical village dwellers. Just like in the 1800s when people were surrounded by farms and a little hamlet. People like this wouldn't go outside their village; their village would be their life. There are still people in England now who have never been to London and they only live a few miles from the place. I don't think we can conclude that they're isolated, they probably mix in very well with the local community. They have to take their grain to market. They just seem to be isolated from the big wide world, not from their immediate world.

Chairman: Do you think we are trying to look at them too much from the point of view of city people imposing our urban expectations?

Rod: Yes, we are.

Hilary: But to some extent he must feel isolated from other people because of his feeling that if his wife dies, then he would have nobody.

Rod: But the people in the city also feel isolated when they lose their loved ones. If you marry and you have a wife who you love, as soon as you lose her you are going to feel alone, aren't you?

Nicholas: I think we're considering the passage too narrowly. I believe what is portrayed here is quite a common human sentiment. I would feel the same as most people, that if you lose someone on whom you are dependent that's a terrible thing. It's not just a matter of functional dependence, it's also companionship and friendship.

When two people are dear to each other and understand each other so well it feels almost as though you have lost half of yourself when a partner is lost.

[*Pause.*]

Chairman: Let's go on from Nicholas's point. Acknowledging that this is a common human sentiment implied in any close relationship, in *this* passage we are dealing with elderly people. Now what are the particular problems in relation to being old and losing a loved one?

Rod: You are then too old to make new ties.

Dave: And old people are not as mobile in their minds as young people.

David: The world has changed around them, and they find it difficult to readapt or look for new friends.

Chairman: That's a very important point.

David: It's hard to tell from this passage whether or not they have any children, but if they did that could help. Having children keeps an elderly person's interest in the world.

Chairman: Or perhaps grandchildren who could be both a source of contact with the modern world, and companionship. Someone said this passage was quite moving.

Brendan: I think the last paragraph is very moving. You can look forward and see what is going to happen to this couple, and that's heart-rending.

Chairman: Is the passage overly sentimental, or is it credibly moving? And if it is moving, how has the author produced that effect without over-stepping the mark into gluey sentimentality?

Rod: I think it's genuinely moving because you can feel it in yourself, you can feel the truth of it. If I was in the same situation myself, I could imagine those feelings to be true. For example, if I were to lose my parents, or a close friend, I would experience this man's fears.

Nicholas: The author uses the technique of describing common events to reinforce the naturalism in the passage, rather than simply using adjectives. I think this helps you; it helps the reader to place himself in the position of the people who are being affected by the events.

Chairman: Could you expand on that a little bit Nicholas?

Nicholas: Well, I could imagine the passage re-phrased with an emotionally descriptive approach, using various words like 'love' and 'fear' and so on. But instead of doing that he's made it a very practical and real passage where many everyday activities are described. They help to set the scene, and are carried over into what's going on emotionally.

Chairman: I like that Nicholas. By using natural images and objects the author has made the reader feel that the old man's emotion is also natural. Just as he reaps the corn and makes bread naturally, his feeling of loss is also natural. Perhaps that's why the group hasn't reacted with any real hostility against this particular portrait of selfishness.

Brendan: I think one could predict that when she dies he'll die soon afterwards. From what's said here one would feel they've both had a very satisfactory life together.

Chairman: Well now, what is the medical message in this passage? Is there something we should take back to the ward or clinic as a result of our reading of this passage?

Colin: I think the passage reinforces the message that the doctor has to have some concern for the family as well as the patient.

Dave: Yes, I think it asks doctors to be aware that people can be combined together very deeply, and, as Nicholas said, losing someone can be like losing half of yourself. The passage asks doctors to look more deeply into the family situation.

Tony: It also asks the doctor to be more aware of the total situation, and how that will affect any decision he is making in relation to his patient. In cases where patients are bonded together as closely as this, it would seem the doctor has a greater responsibility to consider the wishes of the patient's partner. It would involve more joint decisions, I think. If people were joined closely, then probably the doctor should speak to them together. He should treat them more as one.

Jane: And also, if someone isn't progressing as well as you would like them to while they are in hospital, it might be due to reasons other than purely physical ones. It might mean that they are missing their loved ones desperately. Separation in itself can be undermining to health when people are very close.

Chairman: Yes Jane, I see what you mean. I think that's very true in the situation where the wife is in hospital, particularly an elderly wife, and the husband whom she is used to looking after is left at home on his own to do his own cooking and his own washing and cleaning–things which he has never done before. The wife is often very concerned about how he is getting on, and wants to go home earlier than perhaps she would if she didn't have those feelings.

Nicholas: It does underline the fact that when you are treating one patient, you have obligations to the family. In the last medical unit we were in this was often the case. The physician took it upon himself to take care of everybody, not just the patient.

Chairman: What could the liabilities of that be? Are there problems with a doctor taking on responsibilities to the family as well as the patient?

Dave: It can become terribly involved, particularly in relation to time. You can get dragged into a whole family situation.

Brendan: I don't think time is a very good excuse. A lot of people use that excuse, especially when someone is dying. Some doctors use that as an excuse for not talking to patients. I think in the long term it is easier for a doctor to give a wife or husband half an hour of his time, rather than thirty bursts of one minute, especially when the doctor appears to be running away, as if he doesn't want to talk to the relatives. I have seen examples of this recently. On the other hand, someone like Dr Bradley, the radiotherapist, who is a very busy man, always has the time to sit down for twenty minutes or half an hour and explain things to patients. Relatives aren't going to talk to a doctor standing up near sister's desk with the doctor looking over his shoulder creating the impression that he has to be off straight away. They're not going to bring out all their worries in a situation like that.

Chairman: As doctors, we do occasionally get tired and upset and frustrated. When this happens, which aspect of our performance may be pruned away first? When our resources are drained, where are we likely to take shortcuts? Is it in the time spent talking to relatives?

[*General comment*] Yes; that would be pretty high on the list of things that would go. It might be at the top of the list.

Chairman: I think that's true. And I don't say that unkindly, I say it sympathetically. I think as doctors we do get tired and frustrated and anxious at times, and we just want to get right away from the hospital or clinic. We get to the stage where we just don't want to be confronted by another demand or another problem. We don't want to hear the phone ring. We don't want to see a sick person. When we get to that stage, talking to relatives is one of the things we may take short cuts with. I think that this particularly is so when things are going badly, when a patient's deteriorating, or when they develop complications. Doctors look forward to talking to the relatives of patients who are doing well; the converse is not always true. When a doctor is unsure or unhappy about a clinical situation he tends to withdraw. It's at that point that our own resources of good doctorship have to bear their greatest burden. It's when we are feeling lowest ourselves that we have to make that extra effort.

Brendan: I agree with you when you say that. And I agree that when there's a priority of responsibilities in front of a doctor, that talking to relatives is frequently a low one. I still think that it would be a more sensible allocation of time if instead of always running away, a doctor took time quietly to explain and talk without being rushed.

If you did that you wouldn't be looking around the corner for the relative who's chasing you. If you spend time at the start, then you would build a decent relationship with the relatives and it would pay off in the long run. It would give you more confidence in yourself to be able to handle something unexpected or bad later on in the patient's illness.

Chairman: That's a good point Brendan. We will come back in a later session to how a doctor builds a good doctor-*patient* relationship. But your point is very true: that the foundations of the doctor-*relative* relationship are important if one is to avoid that appalling situation where the first time a doctor speaks to a relative is to tell them some really frightening news, or that some complication has taken place.

Well I enjoyed that discussion, you handled it with considerable medical maturity. Let's move on to the next passage which, although a fairly long one, is mostly dialogue, so I think it's manageable. It comes from a story by Luise Rinser, 'An Old Man Dies'.

I stroked Uncle Gottfried's hand. He lay there with his eyes wide open, staring at the ceiling. But I had the feeling that he recognised me, even if only for a second.

'Can't he talk any more?' I asked softly. But I had forgotten Aunt Emily's deafness.

'What did you say?' she shouted, her hand cupped to her ear.

'Please let's go into another room,' I said.

'Why another room? There isn't a fire going anywhere else. We'll have a cup of coffee.' And in a pitiful voice she added, 'But I haven't got a bite to eat in the house. He always did the shopping. I haven't any idea how to do it.'

So Peter went to buy a few things and I whipped some evaporated milk which I had brought along. Aunt Emily made the coffee and continued speaking loudly and incessantly.

'Today is the ninth day,' she said. 'It's the crisis. The doctor thinks he's going to pull through, but the doctor's a fool. You can see for yourself that he has no more resistance. He always drank too much. So that's that.'

She poured the coffee through the strainer.

'Did he ask for me?'

'Yes, the first evening he got the fever.'

'Why on earth didn't you write me right away!' I was angry. She shrugged her shoulders, and then asked, in surprise, 'What good would that have done?'

'Well, my God, maybe it would have helped him a little.'

'Do you think so?' she asked, unmoved. 'He has me, you know' . . .

'How did he get so sick?' asked Peter.

Again she shrugged her shoulders. 'It didn't have to happen at all,' she said. 'But you know how stubborn he is. He had a little cold.

"Don't go out in weather like this," I said. But no, he had to go shopping, and when he got back he had the fever.'

Peter couldn't restrain himself. 'Why the hell did you let him go out when he had a cold? Couldn't you have gone just once?'

She looked at him, hurt. 'Me?' she asked with petulant amazement. 'Why me all of a sudden, when he's done the shopping for forty years?' . . .

The hours came and went. At dawn, Aunt Emily awoke. 'Is he still alive?' she asked loudly. She bent over the dying man, raised the bed covers and felt his legs. 'It'll be soon,' she muttered. 'Soon'. She let the blanket fall back on him, then she shuffled from the room. I heard her fussing about in the kitchen with the stove and the pots and pans.

All at once Uncle Gottfried looked me straight in the eyes and said, with astonishing volume and firmness, 'Be good to Emily.'

Those were his last words; a few moments later, even before I could have called Aunt Emily, he died. The expression of patient melancholy remained on his face. I summoned Peter and Aunt Emily.

'Is he dead?' she asked. And immediately an expression of wild terror was in her eyes, and she began to wail.

She cried uncontrollably, clinging first to Peter and then to me.

But then, just as suddenly, she said, 'So now he's just left me all alone. So that was his trick, just to go away like that. Now I can die for all he cares. He's gone, and nothing can bother him any more.' Peter led her out of the bedroom and into the kitchen. There he let her cry as long and as loud as she wanted.[2]

Chairman: Does this passage produce a different effect on you from the first one?

Colin: It could almost be a continuation of the first passage. Here, Aunt Emily is just so terrified that her husband's going to die that she is indignant when he dies. It could almost be a continuation of the passage on old Henry and Phoebe.

Chairman: Do you feel the same about Aunt Emily as you did about old Henry in the previous passage?

Hilary: No; I don't. *I* see the passages as competely different. I don't think that these two could have ever had the sort of relationship which the elderly couple in the first passage had. There's just too much bitterness here.

Colin: Well if this passage is different from the former one, it could just be because they are further advanced along the path of separation. In this passage one person is actually dying, whereas in the first one old Henry was only considering the possibility of his partner dying. I could imagine old Henry getting like Aunt Emily at a time when Phoebe was going to die.

Hilary: I don't accept that. I think Henry would have been showing far more grief and sorrow than this woman.

Tony: Their lives seem so trivial. The death is in keeping with the circumstances in which they have all been living: the regular routine of getting the groceries, their little fights; and the way they run their lives. Aunt Emily hasn't at all adjusted to the fact he is going to die. She's still preoccupied with the trivial everyday concerns of her life.

Chairman: Do you think she can ever adjust?

Tony: I don't know, but I think she will remain bitter for the rest of her life. She sees the whole thing as just her husband's little game. I feel there is a lot of guilt involved on her part. She thinks it's his last little trick, dying before her.

Colin: I don't think that's guilt. I think she's so terrified she can't act any other way. She just doesn't know what she's going to do in the future.

Chairman: That's a very charitable way of looking at her. What Colin is saying is that the personality being expressed in this passage is not her true personality but one which has been produced by the stress she's facing.

Male student: No, I think she's indifferent.

Robert: It sounds like he's always looked after her, because she says 'Why me?' about the shopping. He's always done it.

Nicholas: I think she's become a totally dependent person. One could also ask why did she become like this? Is this inherent or was it produced because everything has always been done for her? I personally don't have negative feelings towards her, I feel very sorry for her.

Robert: I didn't say I didn't feel sorry for her.

Dave: Yes, I think you've got to feel sorry for her, she's grief stricken because her husband is dying.

Chairman [*smiling*]: You are all being very generous, aren't you? Isn't this just a selfish old woman, an insufferable, intolerable old hag?

Jane: I would like to feel that she had some redeeming features, and that her behaviour was just a way of covering up her inability to cope. But I think the way it is presented–the attitude of the narrator–seems to say that she is a nasty old woman. She is very selfish.

Hilary: Yes, I get the impression that she's carrying on just the same way she had before he got sick. Her behaviour seems more a continuation of her inherent nature.

Rod: I don't think you can tell, from the section we have considered, what she's like at all, and therefore I don't think we can say whether this is her normal personality or whether it's an abnormal defence mechanism. Perhaps she really has an affection for him so she is throwing hate at him because she doesn't want to lose him. She may be talking herself into not liking him so that when he dies she doesn't feel the separation.

[*General laughter.*]

Chairman: That's a very cerebral thought Rod. Is it compatible with the mood of what is being said in this passage?

Robert: Well Rod might have a point, this is just her in a crisis, you can't make a judgement on what she would be like normally.

Colin: One thing which does go against your [the chairman's] argument is the line which says, 'All at once Uncle Gottfried looked me straight in the eyes and said, with astonishing volume and firmness, "Be good to Emily" '. Now, that indicates he had a genuine affection for her.

Chairman: Good, Colin. That does support your earlier suggestion that the first and second passages we have considered are compatible, and that the relationship between this elderly couple did have some depth.

Robert: I don't think that the attitude which she is expressing is all that uncommon under stress.

Dave: I disagree, I don't think this sort of response is ever seen when the relationship between the two people has been meaningful. Let's go back to the previous passage where we had the old man and the old woman who were so totally dependent on each other. I don't think one could ever imagine either of them saying, 'Oh, he's played a trick on me by leaving me alone and dying first.' I can't imagine either Henry or Phoebe saying what Aunt Emily did.

Hilary: I agree with Dave. This seems just too extreme.

Brendan: It's almost like a fungus which is attached to a tree; when the tree dies the fungus gets hostile with the tree for dying. I still feel sorry for this woman. But I don't think she had a very close relationship with her husband. I think the normal reaction of somebody who had a very close relationship would not be the hostility and selfishness which this woman has shown.

Chairman: Well the group's divided. Is there anybody who hasn't spoken who wants to make a comment? Gillian, do you?

Gillian: No, not at the moment.

Colin: On thinking further I agree that the relationship between this second couple is far less close than the first.

Tony: I think Aunt Emily is reacting in a way that is normal to her personality. I think she's lazy. She hasn't perceived his death for what it is.

Chairman: I want to put a question to the group. In your heart of hearts do you believe that the way Aunt Emily is reacting with her selfishness, her crassness, her insensitivity, and her lack of consideration for anyone else, is a response to the stress of her husband's impending death, or that it is pretty much her ingrained personality?

[*General agreement.*] This is her ingrained personality.

David: No, this could be a gross exaggeration of what her normal personality is.

Jane: I think the point where Peter asked her why she didn't go out to do the shopping and she simply rejected the suggestion that she should have done it to save her husband the possibility of deteriorating, shows just how little regard she had for him. I think that's a clue.

Brendan: We're also given a clue by the narrator of the story, he's obviously hostile towards her. I tend to agree with Jane in this. I am sympathetic towards this woman, but I think what is given to us here on the page, is her basic personality.

Chairman: I still don't think anyone has answered Colin's point on Uncle Gottfried's comment 'to look after Emily'. Uncle Gottfried's comment is a charitable one and it shows that he has concern for his wife.

Rod: I think that line ' "Be good to Emily" ' says a few things. First, that she's not acting as she normally does. It seems to suggest that he recognizes that she's treating him excessively harshly because of the circumstances. Second, the words, ' "Be good to Emily" ' don't necessarily imply that there's any great love between them. It would just mean that they've come to live with each other and that they've become coinhabitants of the same house.

Chairman: Could I just read the bit which preceeds the ' "Be good to Emily" ' statement. ' "It'll be soon," she muttered. "Soon." She let the blanket fall back on him'. Now to me, that line is a clear gesture of the contempt she really has for her husband. She let the blanket *fall* back on him. If anyone was ever going to show tenderness, it would be to use the blanket to wrap up the sick person. Could you ever imagine a doctor or nurse allowing the blanket to fall back on a patient? Uncle Gottfried's line is all the more poignant because it comes after that terrible gesture from Aunt Emily. He has almost turned the other cheek.

Tony: It's a very self-righteous turning of the other cheek. If you believe, as the chairman said, that it was at the moment when she'd produced a great indignity on him that he showed this charitableness towards her.

Dave: Maybe he's feeling some sort of guilt. Looking back over his life and seeing the way he's treated his wife, and now he's on his deathbed he's trying to compensate for that.

Nicholas: That's an interesting point because normally it's the relatives who react by saying, 'Oh gosh, I should have done this and I should have done that', when they are confronted with a loved one who is dying. But here Dave is suggesting it is the dying person who is showing remorse for what he hasn't done. Perhaps Uncle Gottfried is feeling a bit guilty.

Stuart: I think this woman really was a rotter. This poor fellow had spent most of his life trying to please her by running out to do the shopping and so on. From that you can gather he must have felt something for her, but that doesn't prevent it from being a one-sided relationship. I think that might be the difference in this case: he loved her dearly, but she just didn't care.

Chairman: That's a good point.

David: Well one thing we haven't thought of is this. People here are saying that she made him do all these things and she's a bitch, but a person can be made dependent by being married to a dominant personality. Maybe he went out to do the shopping because *he* wanted to. Maybe it never occurred to him that *she* might like to do it.

Nicholas: I agree; and ' "Be good to Emily" ', is also very authoritarian. If you look at the lines where Peter led her out of the bedroom into the kitchen, there's a case to be argued that perhaps she's being brutalized into this.

Chairman: Would Aunt Emily be an easy relative for a doctor to handle?

Dave: No, you would have to get the stick out on her!

Brendan: I don't think it would be all that difficult because I don't think she seems to be very emotionally involved. The relative who really frightens the doctor is the one who is deeply involved. I think she'd be very demanding in certain things. But I don't think she would be nagging at the doctor.

Chairman: Does everyone agree with that? [*General disagreement.*] Do you think that a woman like this would actually approach the doctor?

Hilary: No, I don't think so. She's admitted in the passage that she thinks doctors are fools, so I don't think it's likely that she would go and talk to them. Nor would she be likely to accept what they say.

Chairman: Is it a common thing that a relative who has been indifferent during the life of the patient becomes aggressive and demanding towards the doctor when that same person is ill?

[*General agreement.*]

Rod: Yes, I think it's not uncommon to find patients who try to make up for the indifference they have shown during their life with exaggerated gestures of concern when the person is ill.

Nicholas: I agree, they would be the sort of relative who would be ringing up all day and wanting to have a lot of the doctor's time.

Brendan: But that would be more of a nuisance to the doctor than someone who is demanding. I don't think relatives like her (who are just a nuisance) are as demanding as the relatives who keep asking, 'Oh, can't you do anything?' and 'What are you doing?' and 'Can't anything else be done?' over and over again. One of the most damaging effects on a doctor in relation to talking to relatives is if the relative has questioned the doctor's capacity or capability. That undermines the doctor very quickly.

Colin: Perhaps, but a doctor could do a lot for Emily. [*Laughter.*] A doctor could help her get over it and to start functioning again.

Dave: I don't like her. She's a ratbag.

Chairman: There seems to be a fundamental question being raised here. There are many people who in our everyday life we may take a dislike to. When we are away from the hospital or clinic we have full licence to dislike them. If we are at a party, or a social gathering, or at the university, we don't have to put up with people we dislike. On the other hand, there may be some *patients* for whom our immediate response is 'I dislike this person'. Now, do we, in the clinical situation, have the same licence to let our dislikes display themselves as we do in our private lives?

Many students [*talking together*]*:* No, no, that's a different situation ... We don't have that right in the clinical situation.

Brendan: In a professional sense you've got no right to judge anyone.

Chairman: Or if you do judge them, the effect of that judgement shouldn't express or manifest itself in your relationship with the patient?

Dave: Yes, but it's not always an easy situation. If you really took a dislike to a patient, then at some point it probably would affect your objective care of them. But I agree with Brendan's point that professionalism should make us strive to overcome that.

Stuart: I agree it probably *should* help us over-ride our dislike of a specific patient, but I think this leads us on to another point. If a doctor found that he couldn't, in all sincerity, treat the patient free of his prejudices or hostilities, then he should suggest that the patient consult another practitioner. I am saying that there are cases where, no matter how professional you are, you could be so adversely affected by the patient that it would be better for you to send them somewhere else ...

Brendan: I don't think that would be unprofessional because I don't think it's interfering with your professional judgement if you send them on.

Stuart: Look, I am sure every so often there must be one patient who comes along, where the doctor feels that no matter how objectively or independently he tries to look at it, the patient still gets under his skin and irritates him so much that he can't look after them.

Nicholas: But that's not the common sort of patient which doctors are dealing with.

Chairman: Nicholas, I think that comment is irrelevant because Stuart began his comment by saying that it was the 'one in a hundred' or the 'infrequent' patient whom he was referring to. He said that every now and again there is going to be a patient for whom the doctor-patient relationship is so undermined by the doctor's basic hostility or incompatibility with the patient, that it's good medicine and good professionalism, under those circumstances, to send the patient on to someone else. Now to say that that situation is uncommon is irrelevant to the point Stuart was making.

Nicholas: I accept that, but I would also like to say that negative feelings are not uncommon in the hospital and that the majority of doctors don't buy out of cases because they have such feelings against a patient. I think it can be a higher form of professionalism if a doctor can get over that.

Chairman: I agree, and that's a very relevant point too, because if we come back from the uncommon situation which Stuart was describing towards the commoner situation which Nicholas mentioned, we are into an area where this greater demand on the doctor asks him to raise his level of performance to produce something which could be called good doctorship.

This problem of the irritating patient is one point where some people outside the profession might find it difficult to understand what it means to be a doctor or a nurse.

Rod: It's only the very personal prejudices which act when a doctor is looking after a patient. You might have doctors who believe in the White Australia policy, but when they come to treat someone who is coloured, they treat them normally. They don't let it interfere with their professionalism. It's not the philosophical or doctrinal prejudices that are important, so much as the personal ones. It's the patient who irritates you who is more of a danger than the patient who may hold an opinion different to yours on a basic issue.

Nicholas: I think one patient who's very difficult is the one who's failed to take the doctor's therapy, or who's failed to accept his recommendations over and over again, when it's obvious they are the right ones, and through not following them, the patient's health is deteriorating.

Chairman: There are many different sorts of patients who might irritate us. We discussed the problem of the patient who was a 'snob' last week in relation to the Solzhenitsyn passage in which Pavel intimated that he was 'better' than other patients–a point which Gillian took issue with.

I believe that the practice of doctorship is not always the same as the theoretical ideal. People outside and inside the profession try to define the ideal doctor, but we are human like everyone else. Our performance will always fall short of our ideal for a whole lot of reasons which are difficult, but not impossible, for outsiders to appreciate. This is not to say we shouldn't strive to reach these ideals. But as human ability always falls short of human aspiration, it is honest for us to discuss these problem areas and to admit when our performance could be improved.

There's a sonnet of Shakespeare's which I would like us to turn our attention to now. I think it follows on nicely from the sentiments in the two passages which we have been discussing.

Tir'd with all these for restful death I cry,–
As to behold desert a beggar born,
And needy nothing trimm'd in jollity,
And purest faith unhappily forsworn,
And gilded honour shamefully misplac'd,
And maiden virtue rudely strumpeted,
And right perfection wrongfully disgrac'd,
And strength by limping sway disabled,
And art made tongue-tied by authority,
And folly, doctor-like, controlling skill,
And simple truth miscall'd simplicity,
And captive good attending captain ill–
  Tir'd with all these, from these would I be gone,
  Save that, to die, I leave my love alone.[3]

Chairman: Could we look at this first as a poem, and then the message of the poem in relation to the theme that we have discussed so far today.

David: What the poem seems to say is that there are a lot of things which one doesn't like in the world, and that one would like to die to get away from it all. Then the poet says that there is this one thing: 'Save that, to die, I leave my love alone.' The implication is that the poet doesn't want to die because the richness of a human relationship outweighs all of the hateful aspects of life.

Chairman: Good, I think that's a clear paraphrase of the sentiment of this poem.

Doug: Is Shakespeare being cynical when he writes this?

Chairman: What does the group think, is this a cynical sentiment?

Dave: No, I think it is down to earth and straightforward.

Chairman: How effective is the poem in expressing the sentiment that David gave us in his interpretation? Is it a good poem?

Rod: I don't know if this is how it was written intentionally, because I don't understand this sort of English, but I got tired of reading all those repetitious lines; but finally, in the last two lines, which explain it all, the meaning comes through. The final two lines made it all the more striking to me, because I had got tired of reading the repetitious part, 'And this, and this, and this, and this'. As he says himself 'Tir'd with all these, from these . . .'

Chairman: Did other members of the group get tired of those lines?

Robert: Yes, I was bored stiff.

Hilary: I wasn't. I don't think that sense of repetition distracts from the beauty of the poem.

Brendan: Nor do I. I think it makes the final two lines far more meaningful.

Nicholas: This is a beautiful poem. In those lines Shakespeare is building up the whole intensity of the experience of life.

Colin: Those lines clarify what it is he is talking about. The last two lines–the sentiment of the last two lines– would be meaningless without the preceding section.

Nicholas: The technique he is using is, through the very repetitious nature of it, to build up a feeling of anger and indignation as to the injustices of life. I was trying to feel the lines as I was reading them.

Brendan: Every line is just superb. What he has written isn't repetitious at all. In every line there's something different.

Rod: Well, I would like the lines explained before I make up my mind on that.

Chairman: This could be a key point, Rod. Appreciation must be preceded by understanding, unless the poem is so obscure as to be beyond comprehension, in which case that confusion would be a criticism of the poem. But you would agree that we should strive for an understanding of what is being said before we make up our mind as to whether or not we dismiss the sentiments being expressed.

Gillian: Yeah, I think what the guys who don't like it are saying is that they don't understand what the lines are saying . . .

Rod [*interrupting*]*:* Just a minute, I didn't say I didn't understand what he said, what I am saying is that I just don't think there's anything great and beautiful in each line. All I am saying is that for me, it's the last two lines that make the poem . . .

Chairman: Well you said before, and some people disagreed, that the lines which were an inventory of the 'ills of life' were tedious. But let's go back to Gillian and let her finish what she was going to say.

Gillian: I think each line is said in a really beautiful way. Lines like 'And right perfection wrongfully disgrac'd'.

Nicholas: And a line like 'And art made tongue-tied by authority'.

Brendan: Yes.

Chairman: I agree, that's a superb line.

Gillian: I like the line 'And captive good attending captain ill'.

Chairman: Each line seems to embody a philosophy in itself?

Gillian: Yes.

Chairman: Nevertheless, to consider Rod's point, there are certain lines which none of us have mentioned, and I think some lines in this poem do need explanation. So to try and help those of us who feel some of it is unclear, let's go through the difficult lines. 'And needy nothing trimm'd in jollity', now what does that mean?

[*Pause.*]

Nicholas: Excess with more excess on it. Is that what it means?
Chairman: This line highlights Rod's comment that some of the lines are obscure. Let's wrestle with it.
Colin: Well, I'm not afraid to show my ignorance. Perhaps he's saying that one who needs nothing has got everything.
Rod: No, he's saying that somebody who *should* have something has nothing.
Chairman: That's the way I read it: that 'needy nothing trimm'd in jollity' could mean a brave face put on by someone who really has nothing and is in need. Shakespearian scholars discount this interpretation and . . .
Stuart: I agree with that.
Chairman: We can't be dogmatic about it. Now what about the line 'And purest faith unhappily forsworn'?
Gillian: I think this expresses the feeling of being let down, a disappointment, where your trust has been misplaced.
Brendan: It expresses the sentiment where all your ideals come crashing down in disappointment.
Chairman: And the line 'And gilded honour shamefully misplac'd'?
Brendan: It's like looking up to people with titles and honours who you respect.
Stuart, Gillian, and Robert: No, that's not what it means.
Brendan: Well let me explain! The Shakespearian concept of honour, or at least the Elizabethan concept of honour, of something not seeming to be what it is, or what it is portrayed to be, is the way I read it.
Gillian: Does it mean that somebody is fighting for something which really doesn't mean anything, that isn't worthy.
Chairman: The only thing which makes me a little uneasy about that interpretation is the word 'gilded'.
Rod: I agree. It sounds more like the giving of honours (things like knighthoods and so on) to people who aren't really deserving. While the people who are deserving go along without any recognition.
Chairman: Does the group feel that 'gilded' is different from 'golden', and that the use of the word 'gilded' is suggesting that the honour isn't quite the full mint?

[*General agreement.*]

Chairman [*smiling*]: Now what about the line 'And maiden virtue rudely strumpeted'?

Robert [*coyly*]: Well I . . . Well we won't go on with that!

Chairman: Do you understand that one Rod?

[*General laughter.*]

Dave: What about you Jane?

[*More laughter.*]

Chairman: And the line 'And right perfection wrongfully disgrac'd'?

Nicholas: The innocent being called guilty.

Dave: Yes, that's a wonderful line.

Chairman: And now the line 'And strength by limping sway disabled'?

Rod: Well it's almost like when you see cripples, people who may be paraplegic, who are really well-built athletic people in the upper half of their body and then you see their legs and the paralysed part of their body which is disabled.

Chairman: That may be a rather specific reading Rod, but obviously the sentiment of the healthy body being undermined is clear in that line.

Dave: I don't think it necessarily needs to apply to physical limping, it could be mental–like King Lear in the storm.

Chairman: Or it could refer to a government or nation subverted by disloyalty or treachery. 'And art made tongue-tied by authority', what does that mean?

Nicholas: Excessive regimentation.

Brendan: That's a fantastic line. It could mean censorship. It could be the Australia Council censoring art.

Chairman: You could read it literally like that. Is there any other meaning that could be placed on that line?

Dave: You could take it literally, but I think there's a second possible meaning. The whole vocabulary of the art world to me is just totally foreign. I've read lots of reviews in the papers and things that I have seen lying around my own house, and I find them just very, very, hard to understand. The language used to describe the world of art seems artificial. Sometimes you feel almost as though you need an art dictionary to understand what is being talked about.

Doug: In the sixteenth century there were certain limitations on people, particularly in relation to what you could do or say, especially in the Elizabethan court. We might have to read that line in terms of the time that the poem was written.

Rod: It could also mean the sort of thing that happened to Galileo and people like that. Galileo was saying the sun doesn't go round the earth, the earth goes round the sun. And that view wasn't permitted by various authorities. The flat-earth minds would be against Galileo and would make him tongue-tied.

Chairman: Now Rod's put a new interpretation on the word art as signifying the imaginative, the innovative, or the exploratory mind.

Rod: Yes; and also those who change to a different style of art. Whenever a new movement comes into art, the authorities frequently say, 'Oh, that's terrible!' and it takes one hundred years before it's accepted.

David: It could be an outcry against excessive reliance on form. Like people two hundred years ago saying that Beethoven's Fifth Symphony is just a lot of noise, while today we think it's brilliant. The poet might be saying there is too much 'tongue-tying by authority' because they're too concerned with form.

Chairman: You mean the critics are imposing the established order on something new. Is that what you mean?

David: Yes. But it could also mean the artists themselves being straitlaced and controlling their own art works by accepting the form of the day. The artist may not let himself go if he is too controlled by form.

Chairman: And Picasso would be a good example of someone who ran his brush through all of those conventions and wiped them out.

Nicholas: That's what I meant when I said too regimented.

Tony: There is also the effect of the expectations of authority in relation to the artist's performance. 'Art made tongue-tied' suggests the desire to get something out without being able to do so. A frustration or an impediment seems implied.

Nicholas: Yes, I think it does imply an hierarchical structure within which it is impossible to move and express yourself in your own way.

Chairman: Perhaps there is a message in this passage for every teacher and his attitude to the students who are under his care. I think a shy student can be crushed by an authority figure. Such a student feels that he or she doesn't want to speak because they will be made a fool of in front of someone who 'knows'. Now I know that I do this to you at the bedside more often than I wish. I hope that I don't do it so frequently in this session.

Are there any meanings of the word 'art' other than the ones we've considered?

Brendan: Well, I suppose as in 'thou art', it could be a tense change, it could mean 'in the past'.

[*Pause.*]

Chairman: What about the line 'And folly, doctor-like, controlling skill'?

Robert: Hmm, nasty!

[*General laughter.*]

Chairman: You think there's a swipe being made at doctors?

Students [*generally*]*:* Yes, it seems so.

Chairman: Well if it is, it's very unusual for Shakespeare. Alone among the Elizabethan and Jacobean dramatists and poets, Shakespeare had a warm affection for doctors. There are eight doctors in Shakespeare's plays and apart from Dr Caius, in the *Merry Wives of Windsor*, all of them are portrayed with affection. Why this is, I'm not sure. Shakespeare's son-in-law, Dr John Hall was a doctor, and a much-loved doctor. There are reports of him leaving the municipal meetings in Stratford to attend sick patients. No doubt his performance had an effect on Shakespeare's attitude towards the medical profession. So if this is a swipe at medical doctors, then it is unusual for Shakespeare. Shakespeare showed his doctors to be tender and concerned about their patients.

David: Could he just be saying that doctors control things: that doctors are in charge of the situation and control the skills involved?

Brendan: He may not be talking about doctors of medicine. The majority of doctors at this time were doctors of divinity or doctors of philosophy. He may just be criticizing learning–academic learning–rather than the medical profession.

Doug: In Shakespeare's writing in general does he call them 'doctors' or 'physicians'?

Chairman: That's a good question. Now I am not sure. I have a feeling that he does refer to 'physician' in *King Lear*, but as far as I can remember I think in *Macbeth* he's called 'doctor'. I would have to look that up Doug. I'm not sure.

Nicholas: Is he making a differentiation, an early differentiation, between the two sides of being a doctor, one the human side, and the other the mechanistic side?

Chairman: I'm sorry, I missed that. What did you say Nicholas?

Nicholas: Well Shakespeare might on the one hand be very disposed to doctors because of the human aspect of their care, but at the same time badly disposed to them because they often do things which are not particularly effective.

Chairman: I would say that generally Shakespeare didn't criticize doctors for not doing what they couldn't do. He tended to have regard for them if they showed the sort of behaviour which any doctor can achieve no matter how primitive the state of his medical science. Things like humane concern and care, and a basic consideration for the patient.

Let's continue. This section of the poem ends with the line which some of you have mentioned before as being rather magnificent, 'And captive good attending captain ill'. And it leads up to the 'Tir'd with all these, from these would I be gone, / Save that, to die, I leave my love alone.'

Rod, would you like to make any further comments now that we have gone through the lines in detail?

Rod: I still feel that while each line on its own might be good and I could talk about them for hours, just reading it I found I got tired of reading all of those lines before I got to the last two. And that made me all the more appreciative of 'Tir'd with all these . . .'.

Chairman: Well, that's an interesting point. *You* got tired of them and perhaps we were meant to get tired of them because the writer of the poem was expressing the sentiment that it was his 'tiredness with all of these' that made him yearn for death. It may be that your reading is a very sensitive one Rod!

[*General laughter.*]

Male Student: It's a small possibility!

Nicholas: But a poem like this shouldn't be read in a detached way. One has to listen to it as one reads it and enjoy the feeling of what the poem is saying.

Chairman: There are no laws on how people should read poems.

Nicholas: But poems and plays are not written to be static.

Gillian: That doesn't mean to say you can't enjoy them by reading them.

David: But you can't just read Shakespeare through 'zap', just like that! You've got to sit and work out 'What does this mean?' You can't read it like you would read an ordinary novel.

Gillian: Just look how long it has taken us to work out the meaning and the beauty in each line.

Robert: Yes, I agree.

Chairman: Has it been a rewarding activity?

Gillian: Yes, I think so, very much.

Chairman: What does the group feel? This is the first time we have engaged in a little literary diversion.

[*General comment.*] Yes, it's been an interesting thing to do.

Chairman: Now the reason I put this poem in was not for purely literary purposes, but because it seemed to fit into the theme of the significance of 'loss' which is what we had been discussing with the earlier two passages.

Dave: Are we going to get on to that now?

Chairman: Would you like to?
Dave: Well so far this passage has been a bit of an English lesson!
Chairman: Do you object to that?
Dave: No, I enjoyed it very much. But I enjoy the medical aspects of our discussions as well, and I would like to get on to those now.
Brendan: Let's read the Enid Blyton passage now.

[*Wild laughter.*]

Chairman: O.K., we shall.
Male student: Is this Noddy?
Gillian: No, it's from *The Magic Faraway Tree.*
David: Fantastic!

> For a few days the children had no time even to think of going to their friends in the Faraway Tree. Their mother was in bed ill, and the doctor came each day.
> 'Just let her lie in bed and keep her warm,' he said to the two girls. 'Give her what she likes to eat, and don't let her worry about anything.'
> The children were upset. They loved their mother, and it was strange to see her lying in bed.
> 'There's all that washing that I had to do for Mrs Jones,' she said. 'No, you girls are not to try and do it. It's too much for you.'
> Moon-Face and Silky came to visit the children one morning, and were very sorry to hear that the children's mother was ill.
> 'She worries so about the washing,' said Bessie. 'She won't let us two girls do it. I don't know what to do about it!'
> 'Oh, we can manage *that* for you,' said Silky at once. 'Old Dame Washalot will do it for nothing. It's the joy of her life to wash, wash, wash! I believe if she's got nothing dirty to wash, she washes clean things. She even washes the leaves of the Faraway Tree if she's got nothing else to wash. Is that the basket over there? Moon-Face and I will take it up the tree now, and bring it back when it's finished.'
> 'Oh, thank you Silky darling,' said Bessie gratefully. 'Mother will be so pleased when I tell her. She'll stop worrying about that.'[4]

[*During the reading of this passage there was a lot of laughter and good-natured comment, particularly about Dame Washalot.*]

Chairman: Well, who would like to start the discussion on this passage?
Rod: I would like to say one thing straight away about this. Reading this passage makes me appreciate so much more, some of the other passages we have considered. [*Laughter.*] I mean the other passages have said so much more and in a lot less space and words. I appreciate that it depends to some extent on who you are writing

for, but it just struck me reading this just how good some of the writing we have considered has been.

David: I don't know if this says anything about me, but this is the only extract that we have considered so far in the course of which I have read the whole book! [*Laughter.*] To a great extent the passage reflects on the futility of the doctor saying to the patient, 'Don't worry.' The anxious patient who is in hospital, if he is told 'you mustn't worry', worries himself sick. The patient may be worrying because he hasn't got the money to pay the school fees for his children, or that he might lose his job. A ward sister might say to a female patient, 'You mustn't worry about the children'. Well of course she will continue to worry, that's just a meaningless thing to say.

Hilary: It seems to me that the friends and the relatives are showing more concern about the problem that's worrying the patient than the doctor. It is not the actual illness which is the problem, it's the effect the illness has produced. I mean the effect it's having on their life. The only person who isn't really achieving anything in this passage is the doctor. He is just making sweeping statements. It's everyone else who is helping out.

Doug: It says the doctor came each day so it could have been something serious.

Gillian: This is a common attitude to illness: that you have to pad the patient in cottonwool. You have to protect them from worrying about things. Now it's important for doctors to realize that even when they can't do anything for the illness they can always do something about taking away the other worries that the effect of the illness has produced.

Nicholas: I think it points to the fact that in illness the little things you do to keep yourself busy can prevent you thinking about what is going on in relation to your illness.

Colin: It shows that the relatives wish to do something for the patient; in this case the washing. They're helping out. They're an important part of the assistance given to the patient.

Chairman: Is there any other medical point which is being raised by the passage?

Tony: With a stretch you could say it raises the whole area of community assistance in illness. In this case the illness isn't perceived as a burden on the community, it's going to be magically looked after by some fairy-tale fictional person. The things that they can't do are going to be looked after.

Chairman: Just restate the last bit of that again Tony.

Tony: The burden placed on the community by a person's illness is here being looked after by magical people, by a person who won't charge, and who is available.

Chairman: I understand. Now is there, in medical practice, a real-life equivalent of this magical individual?

Gillian: A grandmother might fulfil that role.

Hilary: Or relatives in general.

Stuart: A social worker might.

Jane: The neighbours might help out, council workers, or district nurses.

Chairman: Which specific services are available in society to tide people over short-term problems?

Brendan: The church used to be.

Dave: The church still is in a lot of areas.

Gillian: Meals on Wheels.

Hilary: Yes, it's the practical services like Meals on Wheels.

Stuart: Social workers, I don't think we have given them enough credit.

Chairman: Are there any associations?

Students: Yes, there's Alcoholics Anonymous, Weightwatchers, colostomy clubs, ileostomy clubs, there are lots of them.

Brendan: The colostomy clubs are marvellous in what they do for patients! The members are almost proud of their stomas, or at least their ability to cope with it.

Dave: What exactly do they do? Could I just ask that?

Brendan: They have meetings, and discuss the problems or complications of colostomies and how to handle them. There is a lot of social support and it reduces their embarrassment. They learn to become socially active again. The bag of a colostomy is a bit of a burden and an ileostomy is even worse. Through talking about their fears they realize that other people aren't going to smell it and they aren't going to be disagreeable. It helps them from becoming upset.

Chairman: Thanks Brendan, that's spot on! Colostomy club members will also come up to the ward and talk to patients who are coming up for the operation. They can answer questions openly.

Is there anything else to say about this passage? A female member of the last group said it is a lot of male chauvinistic nonsense.

David: Chauvinistic nonsense?

Chairman: Yes. The doctor is a male, the mother does the washing, the girls accept the task of the domestic duties, and finally Mrs Washalot is going to help out. The male is the professionally qualified individual and the women are the hacks.

Dave: So it should be! That seems fair enough!

Gillian: This is why Enid Blyton was rightfully criticized!

David: She is only expressing the social attitudes which were prevalent at the time.

Nicholas: It is not arguing for, it is, in fact, arguing against it in a way.

Chauvinism implies that there must be an emotional tone supporting this. That's not true at all of this passage.

Stuart: How do you know the doctor was a male?

Gillian: Because the passage says '*he* says'.

[*Laughter.*]

Rod: It could be ambiguous though Stuart!

[*Loud laughter.*]

Chairman: I shall pour out the drinks while you are reading through the next passage. It comes from a short story by Conrad Aiken, 'Silent Snow, Secret Snow'.

> After supper, the inquisition began. He stood before the doctor, under the lamp, and submitted silently to the usual thumpings and tappings.
>
> 'Now will you please say "Ah!"?'
>
> 'Ah!'
>
> 'Now again please, if you don't mind.'
>
> 'Ah.'
>
> 'Say it slowly, and hold it if you can–'
>
> 'Ah-h-h-h-h-'
>
> 'Good'.
>
> How silly all this was. As if it had anything to do with his throat! Or his heart or lungs!
>
> Relaxing his mouth, of which the corners, after all this absurd stretching, felt uncomfortable, he avoided the doctor's eyes, and stared towards the fireplace, past his mother's feet (in gray slippers) which projected from the green chair, and his father's feet (in brown slippers) which stood neatly side by side on the hearth rug.
>
> 'Hm. There is certainly nothing wrong here . . .'
>
> He felt the doctor's eyes fixed upon him, and, as if merely to be polite, returned the look, but with a feeling of justifiable evasiveness.
>
> 'Now, young man, tell me,–do you feel all right?'
>
> 'Yes, sir, quite all right.'
>
> 'No headaches? No dizziness?'
>
> 'No, I don't think so.' . . .
>
> 'What could it be?' This was his father's voice.
>
> 'It's only this curious absent-minded–' This was his mother's voice. In the presence of the doctor, they both seemed irritatingly apologetic.
>
> 'I believe it is something else. Now Paul–I would like very much to ask you a question or two. You will answer them, won't you–you know I'm an old, old friend of yours, eh? That's right! . . .'
>
> His back was thumped twice by the doctor's fat fist,–then the doctor was grinning at him with false amiability, while with one

> finger-nail he was scratching the top button of his waistcoat. Beyond the doctor's shoulder was the fire, the fingers of flame making light prestidigitations against the sooty fireback, the soft sound of their random flutter the only sound.
>
> 'I would like to know—is there anything that worries you?'
>
> The doctor was again smiling, his eyelids low against the little black pupils, in each of which was a tiny white bead of light. Why answer him? Why answer him at all? . . .
>
> 'Oh, no, I think not—'
>
> 'But are you sure, my boy?' His father's voice came softly and coldly then—the familiar voice of silken warning. . . .
>
> 'You needn't answer at once, Paul—remember we're trying to help you—think it over and be quite sure, won't you?'
>
> He felt himself smiling again, at the notion of being quite sure. What a joke! . . .[5]

Chairman: A lot of medical practice is paediatrics. This is the first passage in which we have considered something from a child's point of view.

Rod: It's unfair to say this is a child; from the way the patient is thinking, he's a bit more than a child. I think he would have been out of the Children's Hospital by this stage.

Jane: Well whatever the age of this child, it doesn't matter. I don't think the doctor should be doing the whole of an interview in front of the parents. It is too inhibiting, the child is unable to say what he thinks is wrong with him and he can't convey his worries, or anything like that. That could apply equally to a child or somebody who is an adolescent.

Robert: How about the domineering aspect of his father, 'the familiar voice of silken warning'?

David: 'His father's voice came softly and coldly.'

Chairman: Are you supporting Jane's point of view?

Robert: No, I think the patient is older than she thinks.

Jane: I didn't say anything about how old he was. I said it didn't matter how old he was to the point that I was making.

Rod: I agree with Jane, that, especially in the situation where a doctor is asking 'Is there anything the matter?' he's not likely to get an answer if there's someone around whom the patient is frightened of.

Colin: Medically speaking the whole thing seems quite a joke. The poor boy is stuck up there in unfamiliar circumstances and it's like an inquisition. He's under a lamp, he's asked to open his mouth, he's examined before a history is taken, then the doctor tries to be nice when he can't find anything wrong with him, and then he tries to take a bit of history, while his parents are around.

Hilary: It seems to me that the boy is unaware that there is anything wrong with him. It seems from the passage as though the parents have called the doctor in to find out what is wrong with the boy. I wonder if he has been misbehaving or . . .

Robert: No, it's his absent-mindedness which they have been worried about, and yet when you read it through he doesn't seem absent-minded. He looks at everything around the room with quite a degree of detail.

Jane: I get the impression that the boy has got something to say, but that he just won't say it. 'The familiar voice of silken warning' and also when he says, 'Why answer him? Why answer him at all?' I think from those two lines you can gather that perhaps the boy did think there was something wrong with him.

Nicholas: I don't think he's got a problem. I think he has a secret. You could build a story around this.

Chairman: That's an interesting comment. It would be an intriguing exercise for each of us to continue the story and predict what we think is wrong with this child.

[*General agreement.*]

Nicholas: I think maybe he's found something out and made the mistake of telling his parents part of the secret.

Chairman: Well, we could go on with speculation, but could we come back to what is happening on the page here?

Stuart: Yes, I think there's a good point made in this passage: in paediatrics especially, the consultation is a closed circle and the patient is frequently left out–just as in this case. He's been examined but the only people who have been consulted as to his well-being are his parents and the doctor. Now as the patient is the most important person . . .

Brendan: The passage is also telling us that children are old enough to tell their own story and that the parents at some stage should be put out.

David: You've got to have some sort of reasonable relationship with children of this age. They won't trust you if you are going to be condescending to them. I think it's very difficult to relate to them as a medical student. I don't know just how quite to react to them. I know at a young age I was very cynical towards the school doctor.

Chairman: This is another side of the problem of being a young doctor and dealing not only with old patients (as we considered in the first half of today's session) but also with young people. It takes a lot of imagination to realize what it is to be someone who is not our own age. As doctors, a lot is asked of us in terms of our range of sympathies.

Nicholas: I agree. The passage is asking us to acknowledge that at some stage every patient wants a private moment with the doctor.

You have to sit down with the patient with a closed door to give the patient his opportunity.

Gillian: I think the passage is also saying that most patients can see right through you when you are practising bad doctorship. For example, when you are showing no interest in them at all, or showing false amiability, or sometimes when you just can't be bothered with a patient at all—those moments when you have to force yourself, it must be very obvious to the patient.

Chairman: And what does that do to the doctor-patient relationship?

Gillian: It destroys it completely.

Jane: I would like to make a point, a general point, about doctors being condescending to patients. Doctors should try and realize that the patient is the most important person. They shouldn't act as some god who's going to fix everything and who knows everything.

Tony: It's interesting the way the doctor immediately asked the child to say 'Ahhh' and the child's response to all of this was 'How silly it was' in the sense that what was wrong with him didn't have anything at all to do with his throat. When we are confronted with family problems or psychological problems our tendency is immediately to jump on to the bandwagon of questions and tests. We tend to interpret the patient's condition in terms of strictly medical problems. And so sometimes we don't confront the real problem.

Chairman: Could I turn the argument round now, and say (for the sake of discussion) that you have all been too hard on the doctor and on the parents. Here was a child with whom there was something wrong and the parents were genuinely concerned: there was something mysteriously wrong with the child and the parents were showing genuine parental anxiety.

Rod: I think Tony may have been a bit unfair because fevers and things like that can make the mind confused and the patient behave abnormally. The child just might have had tonsillitis.

David: Yes, you've got to exclude the physical conditions first to see if there is anything specific you can do about them.

Tony: If that's the case the passage shows the difficulty of doing this sort of examination. Because here, if that's the case, the patient hasn't understood and isn't co-operating as a result of it. Something's wrong somewhere with this consultation. The fact that the child doesn't appreciate the relevance of things, if he was sick, is important. I think it's very important with the more perceptive and more intelligent patients to explain exactly what you are doing and why, so that you can generate some trust for your ability to work out their problem and deal with it. An intelligent patient must feel there is some sense behind your approach. Now I don't know what is wrong with this boy, whether it's a family problem or a real illness, but *he* doesn't have that trust.

Chairman: Can anybody give us an insight into what sort of child this is? What sort of world is he living in?

David: He's very introspective in his world.

Chairman: Is it a beautiful world?

Rod: I think it's a beautiful world! There's a lot of colour and awareness; the flames, the fire.

Chairman: The author also reinforces the smallness of the child–the child views the room through the legs and slippers of his parents. An interesting exercise is for adults to get on the floor and look at what the world looks like to a very small child. Just lie on the floor on your back–perhaps at the next party that David throws . . . [*Wild laughter.*] The boy seems to be living to some extent in his own world. He wasn't taking very much notice of the doctor at all.

David: There's a very obvious thing here where he goes through the descriptions of what he saw. He's noticing all the things around him, and yet he seems to be in his own little world. The conversations around him seem to intrude into the fabric of his own world. The conversation seems to be very sudden and violent when contrasted with the flow of the child's own preoccupations.

Chairman: I agree.

Rod: It points out the importance of taking a history before you start examining.

Chairman: Do you think it would have helped in this case?

Rod: If the doctor could have taken a history he might have got the boy to talk and say what the problem was and he wouldn't have needed to . . .

Chairman: Do you think he could have got the boy to talk with the parents there?

Rod: No.

Brendan: Is it fair to ask what really was wrong with this child?

Chairman: Yes. The story has been interpreted as portraying a child who is gradually slipping toward autism with its inner imaginative preoccupations and its distancing from reality. But at the stage of this extract he really could be regarded as just a dreamy child.

Gillian: A normal child.

Chairman: If you like.

It's getting towards the end of today's session so could I just read out to you a poem called 'My Grandmother in the Shower'.

> Cardigan, dun hose and spangled jiffies
> Abandoned.
> Spectacles too.
> Eyes now unseeing,
> the shower begins,
> tepid and gentle
> enveloping the ancient body.

Hands fumbling for baby soap,
or clutching the rail
and looking frail.
Pelican-thin legs swaying
on the ansell non-slip.
Eyes seeping and sagging.
Amazing elephant folds on her buttocks
A shy eroded erotic zone.
One-two up with the breast flaps,
Give them a good scrub.

Talcum whitening the strange grey-pink
of legs of arms of back of buttock folds.
Throw it up the spout and laugh
at the last intrusion.
No regret in the air though,
all convivial and steamy
after the water-purge.[6]

David: That's superb.

Chairman: Is it true?

Hilary: I find it depressing.

Stuart: I think it's natural and to be expected.

Nicholas: It sounds innocent. It's almost as if it's a young person discovering for the first time what old people look like when they're undressed.

Chairman: Is it humorous?

Hilary: No. I don't think it's humorous at all, I think it's very sad. Just the thought of somebody coming to that state is very depressing, for somebody to become so degenerate and decrepit —when you consider what they were.

Rod: But there's no regret in the poem. I think it's just acceptance.

Brendan: And it's very descriptive, I think the last line is important—'No regret in the air'. Whatever is going on the person is just accepting it, they are quite happy with it, there's no anger or discontentment or resentment.

Chairman: Well how would you respond to that, Hilary: that note of optimism at the end?

Hilary: Yes, well, there is that.

Jane: I think it's very natural. And it's vaguely bawdy—that line about her 'throwing it up' and 'the last intrusion'.

Tony: It's not exactly Max Factor's idea of an ideal woman, is it?

[*Raucous laughter.*]

Chairman: I wonder who Mrs Factor was?

Robert: Matter of Factor's mother!

[*Chuckles.*]

Chairman: It's time we finished today!

ESSAY 2

HUMAN ODDITY: A CHERISHED QUALITY[1]

Such and so various are the tastes of men.
Mark Akenside

In Shakespeare's play *King Lear*, there are some beautiful lines spoken by Edgar:

> Who alone suffers, suffers most i' th' mind,
> Leaving free things and happy shows behind;
> But then the mind much sufferance doth o'er skip,
> When grief hath mates, and bearing fellowship.[2]

This moving and compassionate sentiment would be an apt inscription for our profession; for ours is a profession which offers fellowship and support to those who suffer the stresses of physical, mental, or emotional debility; a profession whose members have the unique privilege of hearing the most secret, and sometimes sacred confidences of other human beings; and a profession which has the awesome responsibility of complete trust.

It is difficult to be a good doctor or nurse, for none of us can be confident of achieving the single most important quality for the practice of humane medicine: the ability to see and feel through the patient's senses. It is easier to identify the talents on which this gift depends—imagination, and tolerance of human idiosyncrasy—than it is to capture the quality. Let us consider each of these talents a little more closely.

One of the commonest and least imaginative sayings about our profession is that the best doctor or nurse will be the one who has suffered all diseases. Even the brilliant Montaigne mentioned it in his wonderful essays. Now while one could agree with the sentiment, most of us feel moved to record some protest against the consequences! The answer lies more in Montaigne's own maxim that 'There is no example in Caesar's life which is not in my own'.

Through an exploration of his imagination each doctor or nurse has the opportunity to realize what it is to be someone else—to put himself in the patient's position. And while none of us has an ideal imaginative capacity, a Shakespearian capacity, we all have considerable but largely undeveloped potentials. For while Shakespeare appeared to have in himself the germ of every human faculty and feeling, and could follow them through to all conceivable ramifications, he was, like Caesar and like us, a man. Though his talents dwarf us they also dignify us. Edgar's sentiment touches us because it touches our common capacity.

Another philosopher-poet, Shelley, developed this point even further. He believed that the imagination was the 'great instrument of moral good'. Our capacity for love, and our capacity for sympathy with others, is dependent on our ability to 'go out of our own natures' and to identify ourselves with the thoughts, actions, and troubles of others. 'A man', he said, 'to be greatly good, must imagine intensely and comprehensively'.[3] Perhaps he is right. In any event it would seem to be true that to be a 'greatly good' doctor or nurse, empathy through imagination is absolutely essential. For without it the *art* of medicine is emptied of meaning, and the profession stumbles on the single limb of its learning.

It is true that this idea seems far from the problem of memorizing the myriad branches of the ophthalmic artery, or the mysterious mosaics of molecular structure. But the medical schools seem to take good care of a student's scientific vision—a vision which is every bit as important as the part of medical practice emphasized in this chapter. Yet to emphasize does not mean to exaggerate. I am not asking for that sort of empathy with patients which produces debilitating emotional involvement and destroys objectivity and equanimity. Thomas Mann, in his Nobel Prize-winning novel *The Magic Mountain*, identified this dilemma in a passage discussed by the students during Session 3.

One of the ironies of medical practice is that it is often the patient we wish to do 'best' for who suffers as a result of our extra commitment. A patient who reminds the doctor of someone dear—a close friend or a loved one—and who arouses deep human feelings, may cloud the clarity of a doctor's medical thought. This is why we have a professional convention which recommends that doctors should not treat their own relatives and close friends. There are enough responsibilities without the added emotional stress.

Humane care of patients must have a humane basis, not maudlin sentimentality. Nevertheless there are two dangers in complete obedience to the rule that medical people should be on guard against the emotional aspect of patient care. One is that the emotional element and its influence on the patient's thought and feeling is ignored or neglected, and the other that one devalues one's own emotional response to a clinical situation.

Dr John Brown, in his charming short story *'Rab and His Friends'*, drew this distinction. Medical students, he said, 'get over their professional horrors, and into their proper work; and in them pity as an emotion, ending in itself or at the best in tears and a long-drawn breath, lessens–while pity as a motive, is quickened and gains power and purpose.' It is precisely this power and purpose which comes from the effort of imagining the total significance of a disease process in a patient. For in medical practice, as in life in general, the profoundest insight is furnished not by a painstaking observation of what is separate and individual, but by the intensity with which the whole is comprehended. We must put ourselves in our patients' position.

Such an undertaking for every patient will take time; but if medicine absconds from the responsibility of comprehensive patient caring because there 'isn't time', then the most fundamental precept of our profession is in danger of being wilfully sacrificed. To adopt Shelley's sentiment is to recommend an attitude of mind to medical practice; all the time needed is the time it takes to change one's approach. This habit of mind which asks ceaselessly, 'But just what does this experience of illness, or that intended therapy, mean to the patient?' must make demands on the doctor or nurse. It will remind them that they are special people involved in a unique vocation; it will challenge, frustrate, stimulate, and exhaust them.

In striving to incorporate the ideal of imaginative empathy into our everyday bedside routine, and in trying to make it as instinctive as examining the patient from the righthand side of the bed, we teach our students by performance rather than preaching. Like all tasks which involve delicacies of understanding and difficulties in execution, it can only be achieved through repeated conscientious personal application. It will not come through committee resolutions or faculty recommendations. One cannot study it in a syllabus; there is no exam to pass; no new title or honour to decorate our name; no new college gown to adorn our shape. Its influence cannot be proven by experiment, nor will it add to our bibliographies. Its essence is as indefinite, yet as real, as tender, purposeful, human concern. And its rewards are the same; reciprocal increase in human understanding and human dignity. George Eliot captures this thought well in a passage in which she expresses her attitude to her own work: 'The only effect I ardently long to produce by my writings is, that those who read them should be better able to *imagine* and *feel* the pains and joys of those who differ from themselves in everything but the broad fact of being struggling, erring, human creatures.'[4]

The second aspect of humane medical practice that I wish to stress involves our attitude towards human idiosyncrasy. Frequently what a person does or creates is an extension of their being, and to deny its significance is to deny their personal worth. Doctorship asks us to guard our love for what is special or peculiar about a person from that irritable intolerance which dwells in us all, and to cherish not only the rights, but the individuality of the individual. For just as one man's reality is another man's fantasy, so too one man's mood is another man's character. If we claim an affection for our fellows, we claim nothing unless we are endeared to human particularity. Perhaps it *is* better to hate all countries, communities, and committees, and love David and John, than the reverse. Goethe's claim that 'Personal defects are necessary for the existence of individuality'[5] is simple but profound.

We cannot create tidy classifications of what is approved, expected, or allowed in human behaviour. Human practice, like all other natural growths, eludes the barriers of a system. To precisely describe a human being is like trying to describe the forces of a universe–it is impossible.

Is there something in our medical training–perhaps the intellectual security which scientific tidiness brings, or something in our medical manner or our socio-economic class, which blocks out some of our talent for tolerance of variant human responses and attitudes? When the nature of an individual is out of harmony with society's norm, he is open to a whole range of slurs and scurrilities: he is called weird, full of foibles, idiosyncratic, eccentric, a misfit, an outsider, an anarchist, or even a danger to society. A doctor's covenant disallows the use of such charges against those entrusted to his care.

Perhaps Ibsen was right when he said human beings need a *saving lie*: some fantasy to which we cling as fact and without which our lives would be a terrifying chaos. Perhaps some degree of self-deception is essential to human happiness for all except those rare individuals who achieve an inner sense of well-being through a unique, harmonious integration of their personality. For most of us that 'artificial' state is a futile and heartbreaking struggle. We need to nourish ourselves with dreams of how things could be, or could have been. A man or woman will not permit his or her treasured but unrealized ideal to be offended by anyone. The small human stress caused by the effort of supporting the saving lie is but an atom compared with the mass of mental misery caused by its confrontation or collapse. So much of our self-deception is protection against the pains of our paradoxical and ambiguous human state; and so much of it is expressed as our personal idiosyncrasy, eccentricity, or individuality. To love someone with their faults is to acknowledge our common vulnerability and our common frailty.

Two special writers from the past, Charles Lamb and John Aubrey–both antiquarians–had an almost besotting affection for human oddity and and irregularity. They could be recommended as prescribed texts for any students who are involved in a vocation which aims at an understanding of human nature, or a compassionate view of mankind.

Lamb loved humanity, in particular its unusual shapes and sentiments. His message is not just that human idiosyncrasy and oddity should be tolerated, but that—like rare coins or books—they should be valued for their uniqueness. He did more than merely tolerate, he embraced these strange traits and did not wish to change them himself or see them altered by others. Listen to this report in his essay, 'In Praise of Chimney Sweepers':

> I am by nature extremely susceptible of street affronts; the jeers and taunts of the populace; the low-bred triumph they display over the casual trip, or splashed stocking, of a gentleman. Yet I can endure the jocularity of a young sweep with something more than forgiveness.—In the last winter but one, pacing along Cheapside with my accustomed precipitation when I walk westward, a treacherous slide brought me upon my back in an instant. I scrambled up with pain and shame enough—yet outwardly trying to face it down, as if nothing had happened—when the roguish grin of one of these young wits encountered me. There he stood, pointing me out with his dusty finger to the mob, and to a poor woman (I suppose his mother) in particular, till the tears for the exquisiteness of the fun (so he thought it) worked themselves out at the corners if his poor red eyes, red from many a previous weeping, and soot inflamed, yet twinkling through all with such a joy . . . as if the jest was to last for ever—with such a maximum of glee, and minimum of mischief, in his mirth—for the grin of a genuine sweep hath absolutely no malice in it—that I could have been content, if the honour of a gentleman might endure it, to have remained his butt and his mockery till midnight.[6]

Lamb's attitudes are a delightful illustration of his gentle nature, and his enchantment with human particularity.

About the same time that Lamb was writing his essays, Henry-Frederick Amiel was born in Switzerland. He wrote a remarkable diary, from which the following passage—relevant to our theme—is taken: 'Doctors make mistakes because they are not sufficiently individual in their diagnosis or treatment . . . the principal grievance which I have against doctors is that they neglect the real problem which is to seize the unity of the individual who claims their care.'[7]

John Aubrey's *Brief Lives* is an enchanting series of short biographical jottings. His love of strange human habits appears on every page; and he records many, many anecdotes about celebrated people which are only to be found in the *Lives*. His comments about the great William Harvey are illustrative:

> He was much and often troubled with the Gowte, and his way of cure was thus; he would then sitt with his Legges bare, if it were a Frost, on the leads of Cockaine-house, putt them into a payle of

> water, till he was almost dead with cold, and betakes himselfe to his Stove, and so 'twas gone.
> He was hott-headed, and his thoughts working would many times keepe him from sleepinge; he told me that then his way was to rise out of his Bed and walke about his Chamber in his Shirt, till he was pretty coole, i.e. till he began to have a horror, and then returne to bed, and sleepe very comfortably.[8]

Both Lamb and Aubrey teach tolerance and even love of human individuality. It is a talent which all doctors and nurses must gain if they are to be capable of a sensitivity for all human responses to suffering and grief.

There seem to be massive reserves which a human being can recruit when surrounded by crippling conditions. In many cases the human mind seems to have an almost infinite capacity to cope with adversity. But for others—and I feel they are becoming more frequent—the flight of the mind passes less easily from hurt to hope. They realize that the cure for the greatest part of human miseries is only palliative.

Grief is one human emotion which confronts all members of the medical profession. It is one of the most frequent and individual responses to suffering which taxes our understanding of human nature, and makes difficult demands on our doctorship. It is sometimes frustrating to know how to respond appropriately; when to extend support and when to leave alone. It is often at a time when we need to revive ourselves from a demoralizing clinical event or a draining struggle with disease, that we are asked to speak to relatives and to support them. It is then a great task for us to gain some perception of what the event means to the loved ones of the patient who lies dead, or the patient who is dying. At a time when our own emotions are fragmented we are needed to give support to others who are suffering some massive loss, and sometimes flounder in our efforts to be tolerant of all manifestations of grief, no matter how bizarre, or apparently inappropriate, or insincere.

Patients and relatives have a right to their own individuality in suffering; there is no *customary* or *permissible* response beyond which we should react with shortness or disinterest. We have no right to judge sorrow any more than did Hamlet's step-father:

> 'Tis sweet and commendable in your nature, Hamlet,
> To give these mourning duties to your father,
> But you must know your father lost a father,
> That father lost, lost his, and the survivor bound
> In filial obligation for some term
> To do obsequious sorrow. But to persevere
> In obstinate condolement is a course
> Of impious stubbornness, 'tis unmanly grief,

It shows a will most incorrect to heaven,
A heart unfortified, a mind impatient,
An understanding simple and unschooled.[9]

We cannot advise those stumbling with grief as to what is a proper response. Such an approach would be without human foundation, for there can be no community dictate in relation to a personal emotion or a private sentiment. When patients and relatives are under stress or anxiety, when they are undermined by ignorance, fear, tiredness, or anger, we must allow them the licence of their own individuality. It needs great delicacy of judgement to assess the balance between professional aid and professional abstinence if we are to avoid rushing forward with saccharine sentimentality or absconding with brutish insensitivity. We should avoid crass judgements of what is an acceptable attitude or belief in our patients; for the very strangeness of their response may be the greatest guide the doctor has to the essence of their individuality.

There is an irony in the clinical relationship: good doctorship allows the patient the full scope for his individuality but denies the physician the same right. For if it is true that our private self is the prisoner of our own personality, our professional self—which struts on a slightly more restricted stage—should not be. As doctors and nurses we do not have a licence to *be ourselves* irrespective of circumstance. We cannot react to the actions and attitudes of our patients with the sort of indignation and irritation which is our right when we shed our white coat or our uniform and relate to our family, friends, or neighbours.

A medical life wasted because of unhappiness or discontent is a sad thing, 'As water spilt on the ground which cannot be gathered up again'.[10]

SESSION 3

PORTRAITS OF DOCTORS IN LITERATURE

Chairman: Today's topic is 'Portraits of Doctors in Literature', and perhaps we could start by considering a passage from Sinclair Lewis's novel *Arrowsmith.*

> Martin found the hospital routine slightly dull. Though he developed the Intern's Walk, that quick corridor step with the stethoscope conspicuous in the pocket, he did not, he could not, develop the bedside manner. He was sorry for the bruised, yellowed, suffering patients, always changing as to individuals and never changing as a mass of drab pain, but when he had thrice dressed a wound, he had had enough; he wanted to go on to new experiences. Yet the ambulance work outside the hospital was endlessly stimulating to his pride.
>
> The Doctor, and the Doctor alone, was safe by night in the slum called 'the Arbor'. His black bag was a pass. Policemen saluted him, prostitutes bowed to him without mockery, saloon-keepers called out, 'Evenin', Doc,' and hold-up men stood back in doorways to let him pass. Martin had power, the first obvious power in his life. And he was led into incessant adventure. . . .
>
> But on night duty, alone, he had to face the self he had been afraid to uncover, and he was homesick for the laboratory, for the thrill of uncharted discoveries, the quest below the surface and beyond the moment, the search for fundamental laws which the scientist (however blasphemously and colloquially he may describe it) exalts above temporary healing . . .[1]

Chairman: Who would like to start?

Dave: I think it's basically about the character called Martin who has just graduated and who's doing his internship. It describes the way he feels when he's around the wards: he enjoys his first sense of power. But really, in the last paragraph, I feel that he has a secret yearning, not for the actual clinical side of medicine, but for the satisfaction which he feels he would get from working in some sort of laboratory doing research work.

Chairman: What sort of doctor is he?

Rod: What do you mean by 'what sort of doctor'?

Chairman: What sort of clinical doctor do you think he would be?

Brendan: Bad.

Rod: I wouldn't say bad, I'd say uneasy. He seems to be very nervous with patients. I think this is also shown in the second paragraph where he talks about how he likes having the people looking up to him. In that way he doesn't feel as nervous, but when he's in a hospital, and at the patient's bedside, he feels uneasy. He can't treat a patient as a patient.

Chairman: Brendan, you said he would be a 'bad' doctor.

Brendan: Well, what I really mean is that he's insecure in his role as a doctor. He doesn't know how to do it. He doesn't know how to talk to patients. He's all right when he's wearing the badges of rank and thinks that everyone believes he's tremendous, but he hasn't the faintest idea how to relate to people in a clinical setting.

Colin: Yes; he is secure in the impersonal aspects of the job. He feels safe outside the hospital, and he obviously feels that he's going to be safe in the laboratory. He feels confident walking up and down the ward as an intern 'with his stethoscope conspicuous in his pocket'. But when it comes to the patients, he doesn't feel capable in his relationship with them and he doesn't feel secure dealing with them.

David: It doesn't seem to be all that surprising considering, presumably, he is doing his first-year internship. It's not surprising he feels insecure and lacks confidence.

Chairman: You have seized on this insecurity and lack of confidence.

Gillian: Yes, I don't think it's lack of confidence, I think he's really quite bored with medicine. When it comes down to the basics and he's actually seeing a patient, he doesn't seem to get anything out of it.

Robert: It says here that he's homesick for the laboratory and once he'd 'thrice dressed a wound' he's had enough, and wanted to go on to a new experience. He didn't like the routine work in the ward.

Hilary: I think he fears the illness and the pain that he can't deal with as much as he fears the relationship. He says he feels sorry for the suffering; but then says he sees them as 'never changing as a mass of drab pain'.

Brendan: He's a scientist, not a clinician.

[*General agreement.*]

Chairman: Should he be in the ward as a doctor?

Brendan: No he shouldn't. Not at the moment.

Chairman: Is he honest?

Dave: I think he is, because he says he's homesick for the laboratories, so he's being honest in that respect. Whether or not he's honest with patients is another thing.

Gillian: If he was really honest he wouldn't be there in the ward as a doctor.

[*General comment and disagreement.*]

Chairman: Now Gillian has just said that if he was truly honest he wouldn't be there in the ward.

Liz: That's unfair. I think your own suitability to the ward would be something you would gradually become aware of. After all, he is only in his first year out and he's gradually becoming aware of where his interests and his abilities lie. They appear to be in research rather than in the wards.

Chairman: In relation to Gillian's point I suppose we could ask where should he be next year? Should he come back to the ward or move on to where he feels he should be–to the laboratory?

Stuart: He will probably come back for a second year in the ward, but I feel he should move on to a laboratory.

Liz: I think there's a message for us here. A lot of us go into medicine not knowing what it's really all about. What's going on here will probably happen to some of us too when we get out and find that we don't like clinical medicine all that much.

Nicholas: I disagree with the suggestion that he won't stay as a ward doctor. I think that he's very dishonest. He likes the status that clinical doctorship brings, but yet he doesn't actually like to do the job which earns him that status. I think that, for him, the status will be so important, and the feeling of power so important, that he will go along with it and stay in clinical practice.

Liz: But he could have some status and power as a research worker.

[*General comment and disagreement.*]

David: No.

Dave: It's more a backroom sort of job.

Chairman: Perhaps a research worker has prestige rather than glamour.

Liz: Well, as a laboratory worker he certainly wouldn't be so much in the public eye as a clinical doctor. It's a natural reaction for a doctor to like the power of being a doctor, but I don't think Martin will be there for the next umpteen years. He will go because he won't feel that the sense of power is enough to support him for the rest of his life. He'll get a bit bored with that too.

Hilary: But he might not have the strength of character or the initiative to break away from the wards. Having got this far, even though he wishes to go to the laboratory, and even though he's not enjoying clincial work, he might go on being dissatisfied for years like a lot of doctors you see around the hospital.

Gillian: Maybe he'll learn to enjoy it. He hasn't had enough contact with patients to know . . .

Male student: No.

Chairman: What's your feeling about this: if this young doctor stayed in clinical medicine, feeling the way he does, can he be happy?

Doug: No.

Brendan: If he gets into some sort of esoteric set-up, he might.

Chairman: Is there a moment in this passage where he comes close to any sort of personal honesty? Is there any point where he confronts Nicholas's question of whether he is going to go on being dishonest, or going to face himself with his true sense of vocational self-identity?

David: Yes; in the last paragraph. Where it says, 'he was homesick for the laboratory', and then goes on to say *why* he was homesick for the laboratory. Before that it says 'on night duty, alone, he had to face the self he had been afraid to uncover'.

Chairman: Who do you think this 'self' he was afraid to uncover is?

David: If you'd just spent six years training to be a doctor and you suddenly found out that clinical patients weren't for you, it would be a fairly shattering sort of blow. The feeling that you'd wasted six years would be a bit upsetting.

Liz: I don't see them as actually wasted . . .

David: I agree, I wouldn't necessarily say they're wasted either, but you'd certainly feel a bit worried about it.

Nicholas: He's not worried about wasting his six years so much as the fact that he's seeing himself as a very non-human sort of person. I think that's the secret self who he's afraid to uncover: it's the part of him that can't relate to people that he's afraid of. A sentence of six years is far smaller in comparison.

Chairman: That's an interesting point isn't it: the self that he's been afraid to uncover is the one that says, 'I'm not a clinical doctor.' But that's not to say he can't make a very considerable contribution to medicine. After all we could be discussing a potential Sir Macfarlane Burnet, or Sir John Eccles.

David: Yes, there are so many branches of medicine that it's likely whoever you are you'll find your niche somewhere. Martin would have a very good chance of finding his; if he feels so strongly about the religious nature of research, then he'll do it. He seems enthusiastic about it and that's half the battle.

Chairman: I think David has raised a very interesting point in relation to vocational opportunity in medicine. When you add up all the vocational possibilities available after you've graduated, all within medicine, they really are quite considerable. There are many alternatives to clinical medicine: all of the laboratories, bacteriology, radiology, pathology, computer medicine, public health, administration, and many others.

Hilary: But having said that, even with this diversity of vocational opportunity, the inability to relate to people in general is going to hold you back even if you don't deal with patients. Even if you're in research you still have to communicate with other people at a whole lot of levels.

Robert: A lot of that would be written communication.

Nicholas: There is a stereotype of a scientist who sticks to his laboratory and never gets out of it. He is very good with his tools, and yet perhaps not so good with people and poor socially. I don't agree with this stereotype. I recently had a conversation about scientists in history. You find that the people who have made the greatest contribution to medical science have been the ones who have been good across the whole spectrum of human activities.

Chairman: Nicholas's comment leads us straight on to the next passage which comes from Anton Chekhov's short story, 'A Boring Story'.

> He is sure of himself and his [pathology] slides, he knows the purpose of life and is completely ignorant of the doubts and disappointments that turn talented men grey. A slavish worship of authority and a complete absence of independent thought. It is difficult to make him change his opinions, and quite impossible to argue with him. How can you argue with a man who is firmly convinced that medicine is the best science, that doctors are the best people, and that medical traditions are the best traditions?[2]

Chairman: Well, how does this passage relate to the discussion we've been having?

David: This sounds like a pathologist who lacks the self-questioning quality which the doctor in the previous passage had. It sounds as if he has absolutely no doubt about questions which confront him. Everything is black or white.

Stuart: It's almost as though he's got childish convictions, the fact that he believes doctors are the best people, medical traditions are the best traditions—that seems to be to be just a childish conviction.

Liz: There's quite a bit of that around among doctors.

Brendan: I agree.

Chairman: For what reason? Is it justified?

Students: No, it doesn't seem to be.

Chairman: Well society regards the profession as 'special'—shouldn't we think we're special?

Colin: While a lot of patients do think that doctors are special, and that doctors do know most of the things which are related to their disease, many complain that it's all so impersonal. Most patients feel that the personal aspect of care is lacking.

Rod: If you compare the first two passages, it shows up the difference between the clinical side and the laboratory side. In the laboratory you've only got the slide or the X-ray to work on. It's much easier to be sure in that circumstance. But when you're dealing with humans there is the element of human error. For example, when people tell you they feel pain you can't really be sure they are feeling pain. That makes it much harder to be sure about what you're doing.

Chairman: Are you saying that it's less important for a pathologist, a radiologist, or a bacteriologist, to have a knowledge of 'the doubts and disappointments that turn talented men grey'? Is it less important for them to have human understanding?

Rod: Yes, it's not really related to their job.

Chairman: Do you all agree with that?

Hilary: Yes.

Brendan: It is less important for a lot of specialties, that's the reason certain people go in for them. It's because they can't cope with people that they become a—well I won't say it!

[*Laughter.*]

Hilary: But the outstanding people in those specialities are those who also have that element in them where they can communicate and understand human beings.

Gillian: Not being good at human relationships doesn't mean that you can't be good in the non-clinical specialties. Why should you be critical of someone because they can't relate to people if it's not necessary in their job? Perhaps if they don't get so involved with people they can concentrate better on what they're doing.

David: Perhaps people like Chekhov's doctor make the best pathologists.

Rod: What the author's saying is that when you are a pathologist, you've just got to be sure. A frozen section comes down and you've just got to make your mind up; it is or it isn't!

Chairman: Well, could I put two questions to you? First, aren't there areas in all of these specialties which are uncertain and in the region of doubt? And second, if all other things were equal in terms of scientific or pathological knowledge, who would be the better pathologist—a man or a woman who had human understanding, or one who didn't?

Dave: It's a matter of degree.

Nicholas: Every time a new discovery has been made, the person who's made it has doubted everything in that area which has preceded the discovery.

Gillian: That's a different thing, doubting in relation to a discovery is not human understanding.

Nicholas: It's not only human understanding, the point I'm trying to make is that this applies to any branch of medicine. I think that medicine is such an uncertain science that many doctors just can't cope with that uncertainty and become extremely 'certain' to compensate. So you end up with long lists which can't be argued with. What's wrong with this fellow is that he's inflexible and that's a liability no matter which area of medicine you're in—whether or not it required human understanding.

Chairman: The last three of you who have spoken, Rod, Gillian and Nicholas, have made mention of a particular personality type who has an affection for certainty, and who feels secure with that sort of approach. Leading on from that point, let's now consider an extract from Charles Lamb's essay 'Imperfect Sympathies'. I don't believe this passage says much more than what you've said in discussion, but perhaps the way it has been said is different.

> You never witness his first apprehension of a thing. His understanding is always at its meridian—you never see the first dawn, the early streaks. He has no falterings of self-suspicion. Surmises, guesses, misgivings, half intuitions, semi-consciousnesses, partial illuminations, dim instincts, embryo conceptions, have no place in his brain or vocabulary. The twilight of dubiety never falls upon him. . . . Between the affirmative and the negative there is no border-land with him. You cannot hover with him upon the confines of truth; or wander in the maze of a probable argument. He always keeps the path. You cannot make excursions with him—for he sets you right. His taste never fluctuates. His morality never abates. He cannot compromise, or understand middle actions. There can be but a right and a wrong. His conversation is as a book. His affirmations have the sanctity of an oath. You must speak upon the square with him. He stops a metaphor like a suspected person in an enemy's country.[3]

Brendan: That could be a portrait of a surgeon!

[*Wild laughter.*]

Chairman: Cut!

[*Laughter.*]

Jane: Anybody who's *that* certain would not be any good at anything really. If he's so certain he's never going to admit that he's wrong, and he's going to be wrong some of the time . . .

Rod [*interrupting*]*:* Not necessarily, he could be very good.

Jane [*continuing*]*:* If he's very good he could be in greater danger of making very bad mistakes because people are likely to trust his opinions. If you're a pathologist this could mean that you could make just as disastrous a mistake as if you were a clinician.

Chairman: What are the liabilities and advantages of confidence in medical practice?

Rod: You've got to be confident in a job like this. If you're faltering and you don't know what to do, if you wait around and you don't act, you can't be very good.

Chairman: Good. Then what are the liabilities of that approach?

Rod: Well, you might make a mistake.

Gillian: And if you don't admit it you're liable to make that mistake again.

Rod: He's not the sort of person who's not going to admit he has made a mistake.

Chairman: What does the group feel? Is this individual the sort of person who would admit he's made a mistake or not?

Hilary: I don't think he would.

Stuart: He's the sort of person who would say, 'I have made a mistake', but that's all he would say.

Robert: Yes, that's just the sort of person he sounds. It says here 'his morality never abates', which means that he is probably very moral.

Chairman: It *does* say 'that his morality never abates' but we are not quite certain what that morality is!

Liz: It says here that 'Surmises, guesses, misgivings, half-intuitions (and so on) have no place in his brain or vocabulary'.

Rod: Yes, but once he's done something and he realizes he has made a mistake, I think he'd admit it and that would be that.

Nicholas: Just to answer Rod's point, I think there's an issue here. It's quite possible to act quickly and yet to act blind to all of the other possibilities. But even if you are acting swiftly, I still think it's wise to know that there are areas which are dubious in what you're doing. You may have to go back on what you've done, and if you don't . . .

Rod [*interrupting*]*:* But this doesn't say that he's not dubious.

Hilary: Yes it does!

Liz: It does say he doesn't doubt . . .

Rod [*raising his voice*]*:* Just a minute . . .

Chairman: Could I ask a question? Given that there are some areas of medicine where there are clear answers, how would this man face those areas of medical practice where there are no absolute answers?

Robert: I think he'd do very badly.
David: Yes, he'd shy away from them.
Gillian: I don't think he'd get involved with that type of thing.
David: I can't see this man as a psychiatrist!

[*General laughter.*]

Chairman: In which areas of patient care would he be deficient?
David: Any part of medical practice which involved counselling.
Gillian: Yes, I agree.
Liz: And on any aspect of diagnostic thought, if he was going to make a decision and stand by it he'd be a disaster, because that needs flexibility. If he'd made up his mind about a diagnosis on the first day and the whole clinical situation changed the next day, I think he'd struggle to change his mind and alter his thinking. I just don't think he'd be flexible enough to change his mind.
Dave: The decision to treat a lot of things, for example the various cancers and so on, where there is no clearly established best method of treatment, would be a difficult area for him. In that area you can't afford to be as inflexible as this bloke seems to be. Also, you might have to take into regard the family, the social effects, the economic effects, and the human effects, all would need to be considered. This sort of person wouldn't be very good at all.
Jane: He'd be the sort of doctor who would come and tell the patients what they had and then just walk off.
Gillian: I don't think he'd understand the patient's reaction to illness; he'd find it very hard to understand other people's feelings and reactions.
Chairman: The sort of thing we were discussing last week: the ability of a doctor to put himself in somebody else's position.
Gillian: Yes; he just couldn't do that because he's so obsessed with the way *he* feels and thinks.
Dave: He wouldn't understand anyone who reacted at all differently from the way he would react.
Chairman: How damning a quality is that in relation to doctorship?
Gillian: That's just very damning in a certain type of doctor, because it's so important for clinical medicine. But I suppose he could be a very good doctor in another field, where he doesn't have to have any contact with patients at all.
Chairman: Does the group agree with Gillian's point of view that the further away from patients this fellow is the better?
Nicholas: No, because he could be good for a certain sort of patient . . .
Chairman: But surely that's just the point that's been made. Gillian has just said that the patient would have to be like him, otherwise he wouldn't be able to relate to them. As the majority of patients

wouldn't be like him, his satisfactory doctor-patient relationships would be very few.

Stuart: Yes, most patients would be sick for a start, which would make them very different to him. He'd have very little perception of what they were experiencing.

David [*smiling*]: If he had a very sensitive resident he might not be such a bad consultant.

Hilary: Well I don't know, he's not the sort of person who would attract a sensitive resident to his ward.

Chairman: What sorts of things influence a student or resident when they are deciding which consultant to join?

[*General comment*] The personality of the consultants, that's the most important thing if all students could have their way—but it depends on how you do in your exams.

Chairman: Rod, do you want to say something more?

Rod: Well, what I want to say is whether or not he would be a good doctor would depend on the decisions he made. Because he could make the right decision every time if he had a wealthy experience.

Chairman: How can he make the right decision all the time when many of the areas of medicine we are dealing with have no *right* answer?

Rod: Well therefore he hasn't made a wrong decision has he?

[*General groan.*]

Chairman: No, I meant in relation to his approach to a question which is problematical. For example on a doubtful therapeutic area, or a human issue question, or an ethical question where there is no absolute answer. Wouldn't he rigidly adhere to one side of a two-sided argument?

Hilary: I think the worst thing about this fellow would be that he wouldn't be able to take advice from anyone. In any matters of any importance he would just act on his own decision.

Chairman: How important is the quality of 'being able to take advice' for doctorship?

Dave: Incredibly important.

Robert: Absolutely essential.

Hilary: To be able to learn from somebody who has had more experience or more understanding of a clinical situation is essential to good medical practice; so is the ability to interact with other people on your level so that you can gain from each other.

Chairman: I think Hilary's point is an excellent one. A recognition of the point of our own abilities beyond which we are uncertain or inadequate, and our ability to ask the advice of more senior people in the profession, is so fundamental to the practice of good medicine. *There is always someone above you in medicine to whom you can turn for advice.*

Let us now change our tack a little bit and consider a clinical portrait of a doctor. This is a new passage. It was suggested to me by Jane at the end of last week's session and I am glad it fits in nicely with this week's topic. It's from Simone de Beauvoir's novelette or short story 'A Very Easy Death', which I believe refers to the death of her mother.

> Dr T, who was looking after Maman's general condition, came to see her while I was there.
>
> 'It seems that you eat too little?'
>
> 'I was depressed this summer. I didn't have the heart to eat'.
>
> 'You found cooking a nuisance?'
>
> 'What happened was that I made myself little treats, and then I left them'.
>
> 'Aha. It wasn't laziness, then. So you made yourself little treats?'
>
> Maman concentrated. 'Once I made myself a cheese souffle: after two spoonfuls I couldn't eat any more.'
>
> 'I see,' said Dr T, with a condescending smile.
>
> Dr J, Professor B, Dr T: neat, trim, shining well-groomed bending over this ill-kempt, rather wild-looking woman from an immense height: great men; bigwigs. I recognised that piddling self-importance: it was that of the judges on the bench when they have a man whose life is at stake before them.
>
> 'So you made yourself little treats?' There was no reason to smile while Maman was searching her memory with trustful willingness: it was her health that was at stake. And what right had B to say to me 'She will be able to potter around again'? I objected to his scale of values. I bristled when the privileged classes spoke through my mother's mouth; and I felt wholly on the side of the bedfast invalid struggling to thrust back paralysis and death.
>
> On the other hand I did like the nurses; they were linked to their patient by the extreme closeness of those necessary tasks that were humiliating for her and revolting for them, and the interest they took in Maman did at least have the appearance of friendship. Mlle Laurent, the physiotherapist, could raise her spirits, give her a sense of security and calm her; and she never assumed any superiority.[4]

Stuart: This represents the attitude of the relative of a dying woman to the various people who work in the hospital: the doctors, the professors, the nurses, the physiotherapists, and so on. The passage is a generalization, and the daughter is pointing out that the doctors are aloof and condescending. She believes that the nurses are the only people who seem to have any human interest in her mother.

Liz: I think this passage makes a really good point. That is, that the nurses do have a lot more contact with the patient than the doctors.

The passage contains a marvellous line: the nurses 'were linked to their patient by the extreme closeness of those necessary tasks that were humiliating for her and revolting for them'. I think that's so true. The nurses do get a lot closer to their patients because they go through a lot more with them. But I disagree if we're going to generalize that what she feels about doctors is always true. I think it might have been true that they were condescending, but I think there're a lot of doctors who aren't.

Chairman: She hasn't just said that they are condescending. She has itemized some of the things which have irritated her. What are they?

David: She thinks that the doctors are talking down to her mother. It upsets her when the doctors tell her mother that 'she will be able to potter around again'. They obviously don't think that what her mother has been doing with her life is very important.

Brendan: It's interesting that in this passage the *mother* has adopted the role of 'trustful willingness' towards the doctors who are showing this opinionated self-importance, whereas the *daughter*, who seems more sensitive to the way they're treating her, is the one who's reacting against it. I think that's quite often the case, especially on a ward round when an occasional person mistreats a patient. For example, occasionally I react against the way I see a patient being treated, but the patient concerned is perfectly happy to be treated this way. Some of them don't seem to mind at all, as in this case; often it's somebody else reacting on their behalf.

Chairman: Do you think these doctors may have been exploiting that trust and simplicity of the mother? Or do you think they would treat all patients the same irrespective of how accepting they were?

David: I think this is probably the way they talk to all patients. I don't think they realize they are condescending. The daughter is probably younger than the doctors, who are most likely to be of the same generation as the mother. Brendan was saying that often patients don't seem to mind when doctors are treating them badly, I mean in a condescending fashion. Now it seems to me that often older patients have a concept of what the doctor-patient relationship is like which might outrage people of our generation.

Chairman: Good. Now what else in this passage portrays behaviour which may have irritated the patient's daughter?

Gillian: All of the doctors standing around the bed 'at a height' with the poor patient down in the bed.

Nicholas: It's more than just and inequality in physical position, there's also an inequality in class: the doctors somehow being gods in this particular situation with the patient totally at their mercy. Not only that, but the patient wholly accepting this situation. As the passage says it's somewhat like a prisoner in the dock who may have physical chains, but the patient here has the chains of her illness.

Liz: Another point is that they're well-groomed and she is ill-kempt.

Brendan: I think their whole manner of speaking to her is bad. ' "So you made yourself little treats?" '

Chairman: Yes; and the patronizing phrase before that: ' "It wasn't laziness then." '

Gillian: I agree, that's such an easy attitude to take in relation to patients.

Hilary: The comparison later on also highlights the doctor's performance. In the last line she says of the physiotherapist, 'she never assumed any superiority' from which the reader can assume that the doctors did.

Chairman: Is this a fair passage, is it well balanced?

David: I think one has to be aware of de Beauvoir's ideological prejudices here. She's hardly likely to be the sort of person who would approve of a dominant doctor-to-patient relationship.

Chairman: Does she do anything in this passage which suggests that she is being fair?

Rod: I think in the last paragraph where she expresses her feelings in relation to the nurses: she says the nurses give her mother most time, and the physiotherapists next, and then the doctors last. She implies the doctors came around for three minutes and that's all.

David: Yes, but she doesn't exactly give any reasons for why the doctors behave the way they do, and the reasons why doctors can only be there for three minutes, she just presents the facts without looking at the basis for them as far as I can see. I think it's understandable that the nurses can spend so much time with the patient and that the doctors can't.

Liz: Oh, it's much more than that! I think it's the doctors' manner which has been irritating here.

Brendan: Yes. You can spend only three minutes with a patient and be kind and decent and do a lot more than just stand around with indifference or condescension. You can do a lot more than just stand there preening yourself in front of them. That's the sort of description she's put forward and that's what irritated her. Now this isn't generally true, but it's quite often true. It's not hard to find examples of doctors behaving like this.

David: I don't want to defend the doctors' attitude here because I don't think it is good, but I don't think this is a fair look at it.

Brendan: Not in general, but you can find the example portrayed here anywhere.

Jane: I think where she says that she 'bristled when the privileged classes spoke through my mother's mouth', she sees what's going on from her mother's point of view. The doctors don't.

Nicholas [*speaking more loudly than usual*]: Just going back to David, why should this be a 'fair and balanced' passage? Why should the excuses which produce such terrible human relationships be stated? Now why shouldn't this passage, which presumably was a real event, just be stated? I mean excuses don't really excuse what happened. They may explain it, but that's different.

David: The mother didn't seem to worry about it very much. I think that's very important.

Rod [*to Nicholas*]: Why should you get so upset about how the doctors are treating the mother when the mother thinks it's normal?

Nicholas: Because . . .

Rod [*raising his voice*]: The doctors probably *do* know more about her disease than the daughter does. And the doctors *do* know more about the disease than the physiotherapists, so they have probably got a right to think that they do know more. Why should you get so uptight?

Nicholas: Because I don't think the patient is always the best observer in this situation.

David, Rod, Nicholas, and Liz [*all trying to talk together*].

Nicholas [*with raised voice*]: As long as the patient is happy we can do anything to the patient? Is that it? Nobody's allowed to come from the outside and say perhaps, well maybe the patient is happy but this may not be the best thing for the patient?

Chairman: Rod, could I put a question directly to you? Have you been in the situation where you have seen a doctor performing at a level which you would regard as anything but distinguished, and the patient, either through elderliness, debilitation, or youth, or even through lack of intelligence, hasn't been aware that the performance has been shoddy? Under those conditions have you been critical of that sort of performance?

Rod: Well, er yes, well er I don't like it, but I don't think there is any point in standing up and throwing spears about it. I think you probably should accept it and just try and do better yourself.

Chairman: But you would be critical of it?

Stuart: That's entirely another thing, you're talking about medical performance, in other words if somebody did a lousy marrow biopsy and made a big mess of it . . .

Chairman: No, I wasn't referring to specific medical or surgical techniques, I was referring to human performance.

Stuart: Well I think there's a difference between a doctor who treats somebody badly, and because the patient doesn't understand they're being treated badly, they don't react against it, and the sort of thing we've got here, where the doctors are taking liberties because they believe they are in a position to be condescending towards the patient.

Chairman: I don't want to labour the point but I was trying to ask Rod if he was in the position of an outside observer (as was this woman's daughter in relation to the doctor-patient relationship), would he get indignant on observing maltreatment.

Liz: In what way do you mean 'maltreatment?'

Chairman: In the way portrayed in this passage. Phrases like ' "It wasn't laziness, then" '; ' "So you made yourself little treats?" '; 'condescending smile'; gazing over her 'from an immense height'; 'great men'; 'bigwigs'; 'piddling self-importance'. There seems to be an undertow of patronization towards the patient all the way through the doctors' performance.

Brendan: The only reason this woman is happy is that she thinks this is what it is her lot to get. If someone treated her more kindly then she may get a lot more dissatisfied with what many people in the group have seized upon as satisfaction and therefore the justification for what's been going on. Now, I think we should demand that she should be treated better. I mean, just because she thinks she's happy–if you see something which is grossly wrong, you don't just sit back because the person doesn't appear to be upset about it. You get to the situation where those people who demand, get, and those who don't demand, suffer.

Chairman: So you're on the 'Nicholas' side of the argument?

Brendan: Yes.

Nicholas: Look, I quite agree with Rod that you don't have to jump up and down on the bed when you see something similar to this. The idea is, as Rod said, that we are here to learn and that we should recognize this as bad and learn from it. So I totally agree with him that the main message is for us not to behave the same way.

Chairman: Good. I agree with Nicholas. That point is the key one. The message for us is to identify the way we are not going to perform.

There's a marvellous phrase in here that Liz seized upon earlier in this discussion. Every now and again a phrase jumps out of the page and confronts us with its sheer truth, and I would like to read this one again. 'On the other hand I did like the nurses; they were linked to their patient by the extreme closeness of those necessary tasks that were humiliating for her and revolting for them'. It is well to remember that every time you are feeling revolted by some medical task, the patient is usually feeling humiliation.

That discussion leads us straight on to another passage, the one from Somerset Maugham's novel *Of Human Bondage*.

> From commerce with students and poor people he had the patronising air, and from dealing always with the sick he had the healthy man's jovial condescension, which some consultants achieve as the professional manner. He made the patient feel like a boy confronted by a jolly schoolmaster; his illness was an absurd piece of naughtiness which amused rather than irritated . . .
>
> Dr Tyrell came in with quick movements and a happy breezy manner. He reminded one slightly of a clown leaping into the arena of a circus with the cry: Here we are again. His air seemed to

indicate: What's all this nonsense about being ill, I shall soon put that right.[5]

Chairman: Could I ask first what are the advantages of a doctor who has this sort of personality and approach?
Rod: He won't get depressed about problems he comes up against. He's always got an atmosphere about him that will cheer up the patient.
David [*reading*]: 'His air seemed to indicate: What's all this nonsense about being ill, I shall soon put that right.' If he feels that confident it will make the patients feel confident.
Hilary: I think his attitude might protect him against any threatening situation which would arise. If he didn't have this light attitude he might . . .
Dave: Maybe this attitude is some sort of cover-up for his own lack of confidence. Perhaps he's trying to put up this particular front so that he doesn't make the patient feel that he's lacking confidence.
Chairman: Now what are the disadvantages of this particular temperament in a doctor?
Jane: It might not appeal to all the patients. Some of them could be very worried about their illness, and they might think that he's unsympathetic if he is always jovial.
Brendan: A patient couldn't approach this sort of bloke. If somebody comes up to you and says, 'Good-day, how are you?' and slaps you on the back and smiles, it doesn't make it easy for a patient to say, 'I'm worried about my sex life', or something like that! You'd have the feeling that the patient just wouldn't get a go.
Chairman: So the more delicate the task clinically, the worse this doctor would perform?
Many students: Yes.
Dave: You can't afford to have a flippant manner when you're dealing with patients.
Hilary: It would depend a lot on the severity of the illness. If it is something mild or embarrassing the patient might enjoy this happy attitude to help them get over the situation. But if it was something very concerning and worrying, or life-threatening, patients are not going to appreciate this attitude.
Liz: Yes, I agree with what Hilary said. There is an occasional place for this approach to patients. It could be quite reassuring for a kid.
Colin: A patient being looked after by a doctor like this, just might wonder, 'Did he hear what I said? With all his laughing and carrying on, does it mean anything? Have I said something stupid?'
Chairman: Inappropriate smiling was one of the things which the daughter in the previous passage disliked.
Rod: On that point, don't you think it's a worse condescension if, when a patient is saying something the doctor looks solemn and

goes, 'Tut, tut, tut!' I think sometimes a smile is better than that fierceness. A smile doesn't alarm the patient as much as a grave look. Hilary said that if a patient was gravely ill this attitude would be bad. I think a serious-looking doctor can do damage in that situation as well. If the doctor occasionally has an off-hand attitude, it might suggest to the patient that he has treated this sort of thing a lot of times before, and it might give the patient confidence.

Dave: But some patients might look at it exactly the opposite way and think that he's not taking their problem seriously.

Liz: Isn't it better to be non-committed rather than to be umming and ahhing all the time, or smiling? Isn't it better to show no emotion?

Nicholas: You don't necessarily have to eliminate emotion, you just show concern.

Liz and Robert [*trying to speak together*].

Chairman: Nicholas has made the point that we can always show concern. Now is this doctor portrayed here, Dr Tyrell, showing concern? [*Reading*] 'From commerce with students and poor people he had the patronising air, and from dealing always with the sick he had the healthy man's jovial condescension'?

Brendan: I don't think he's concerned really, he's just doing his job. He's not putting himself up as a sensitive receptor to people's problems.

Gillian: He couldn't satisfy their needs in any way.

Colin: The personal element seems to be lost.

Hilary: It interests me that a lot of nurses behave like this and the patients really appreciate it. You know, the nurse who bounces in and says, 'How are we this morning, Mr Smith?' and 'Have you been a good boy today?' The patients seem to really like it from the nurses. They seem to appreciate that a nurse can be cheery about her work, even though it's demanding and sometimes unpleasant. Some patients might look on the doctor the same way.

Doug: That's all very well from the nurses, but a patient who's very ill is looking to the person who they think knows something about what is going on. They don't want a childish attitude from their doctor.

Gillian: When a patient wants to talk to someone about something they're worried about, it's the doctor they turn to, not the nurse.

Robert: Well if I was sick in bed I certainly wouldn't be upset about a nurse coming to cheer me up!

[*Racuous laughter with a few indecipherable comments.*]

Robert: You know, I mean, I wouldn't object if they were coming in to give me a quick back rub or something.

Chairman: Did you mean a male nurse?

[*Raucous laughter again.*]

Stuart: There are two sides to this story. Dr Tyrell reminds me of a classic family G.P. I once knew. The sort of character who bounces in on one foot, especially with children, and who says, 'Oh what's the problem'. For children this seems to work quite well.

Chairman: So the line 'He reminded one slightly of a clown leaping into the arena of a circus' is a good one in relation to children?

Stuart: Yes, it's a very appropriate line. But you have to be able to adapt for different people. In each situation I think it's a matter of having enough insight to decide what exactly your patient requires. And if he requires you to bounce on one foot, then that's what you give him, and if he requires you to show serious concern, well that's what you should do.

Rod: I think this jovial sort of attitude deals well with the organic problem, but when a patient has only got a functional problem, or a psychiatric or psychological problem then . . .

Chairman: I don't like that particularly . . .

Gillian: Neither do I.

Chairman: I would call them human problems.

Rod: Talking to a patient's wife and explaining to her that her husband's got leukaemia is a psychological problem. But if someone has a broken arm, well that's just straightforward.

Chairman: Do you all agree with this separation Rod's made between psychological and organic?

Gillian: No, you can't separate them.

Brendan: No, certainly not.

Rod: I'm not trying to separate them. They could be going on at the same time. They're different.

Brendan: I think you've just got to judge each situation. You couldn't go up to a patient and say, 'You're going for an operation tomorrow, ha! ha! There's a 90-per-cent chance that you'll die as a result of it, ha! ha!' We are talking about conversing with patients here, we are not talking about doing lieno-renal shunts. Whether or not it's organic, the patient's got fears and worries.

David: It's getting to the stage where we are painting this guy Dr Tyrell as some sort of buffoon. Now that's not right.

Brendan: But he is!

David [*raising his voice*]*:* He is not! Now I don't like bringing the novel into this, but I think Somerset Maugham thought that this guy was one of the best doctors in the whole book–if I recall it correctly.

Brendan: No he didn't . . .

David: The second thing is . . .

Brendan: This is the Outpatient doctor; he was a hopeless bastard . . .

David: Anyway, the thing that nobody's picked out is that it is all very well to say this is a bonzer way to deal with kids, but it says in the first line, from dealing 'with *poor* people he had the patronising air'. Well, as far as their health was concerned, poor people in London at the turn of the last century were perhaps a bit like children, and this attitude might have gone down really well.

Chairman: That could be true, but it didn't go down well with the author.

Brendan: And the student in the book didn't like this doctor at all.

Chairman: We have considered some passages which portray doctors critically. Let's now consider a passage which does the opposite. It's a poem called 'On the Death of Dr Robert Levet' written by Samuel Johnson. This poem is thought by some to be—no, I won't spoil your reading of it by telling you what other people think of it! Let's just read it and see what *you* think of it.

Condemn'd to hope's delusive mine,
As on we toil from day to day,
By sudden blast, or slow decline,
Our social comforts drop away.

Well tried through many a varying year,
See Levet to the grave descend;
Officious*, innocent, sincere,
Of ev'ry friendless name the friend.

Yet still he fills affection's eye,
Obscurely wise, and coarsely kind;
Nor, letter'd arrogance, deny
Thy praise to merit unrefin'd.

When fainting nature call'd for aid,
And hov'ring death prepar'd the blow,
His vig'rous remedy display'd
The power of art without the show.

In Misery's darkest caverns known,
His useful care was ever nigh,
Where hopeless anguish pour'd his groan,
And lonely want retir'd to die.

No summons mock'd by chill delay,
No petty gain disdain'd by pride,
The modest wants of ev'ry day
The toil of ev'ry day supplied.

*Officious = dutiful

His virtues walk'd their narrow round,
Nor made a pause, nor left a void;
And sure th' Eternal Master found
The single talent well employ'd.

The busy day, the peaceful night,
Unfelt, uncounted, glided by;
His frame was firm, his powers were bright,
Tho' now his eightieth year was nigh.

Then with no throbbing fiery pain,
No cold gradations of decay,
Death broke at one the vital chain,
And free'd his soul the nearest way.[6]

Chairman: Dr Robert Levet was an unqualified doctor who received most of his medical education by working as a waiter in a coffee house frequented by physicians. He was completely unqualified, as were most of the doctors who looked after the poor at that time. He was a personal friend of Dr Johnson, and when Levet died, Johnson wrote this elegy. What do you think of it?

Brendan: I would very much like to be like Dr Levet. It's a wonderful poem.

Rod: In relation to the previous passages we have been reading, the line 'The power of art without the show' is very important. Here is this fellow who is doing all that the other doctors did, but without any of the show, or any of the aura, or any of their 'big-headedness'.

Gillian: The poem is almost a summary of the ideal doctor. It's easy to understand—not like the Shakespeare last week.

Robert: It's very beautiful.

Colin: I think the poem talks of a doctor who is very honest and very dutiful. Very much a man of compassion towards his patients.

Doug: It sounds as though even God has rewarded him by giving him a very easy death. It's almost as if he has been appreciated by everybody.

Brendan: I like the third stanza. 'Yet still he fills affection's eye, / Obscurely wise, and coarsely kind; / Nor, letter'd arrogance, deny / Thy praise to merit unrefin'd.' I really like that. 'Obscurely wise, and coarsely kind' is brilliant.

Chairman: That's a very famous line. What does the second couplet in that stanza mean?

Brendan: Well, the qualified doctors here are referred to as 'letter'd arrogance'.

Dave: The lines, 'officious, innocent, sincere, / Of ev'ry friendless name the friend' is a lovely line to be spoken of a doctor.

Rod: I like the first stanza—a phrase like 'hope's delusive mine'. You think of 'hope' as a rather long tunnel, along which we all travel. Many of these lines contain a whole philosophy.

Chairman: A line I particularly like is the line 'No cold gradations of decay'. Haven't we all seen, in incurable or very ill patients, that terrible disintegration as a patient moves towards death.

Gillian: I like 'No summons mock'd by chill delay, / No petty gain disdain'd by pride, / The modest wants of ev'ry day / The toil of ev'ry day supplied.'

[*Pause.*]

Chairman: We won't destroy the beauty of the whole by dissecting the poem too closely. Could we have a look at another short poem? It's an extract from a very long poem written by George Crabbe who was a doctor and a poet. It comes from his poem, *The Village* in which he portrayed the lawyer, the preacher, etc., and also a quack doctor.

Dave: Dr Moore, what were you going to say about Dr Johnson's poem before we started to read it—when you stopped?

Chairman: I was going to say that the poem of Dr Johnson's is regarded by some, for example the present Professor of Poetry at Oxford University, Professor John Wain, to be the finest elegy in the English language. In many ways the poem represents the best in Augustan poetry where the job was not so much to say something new, but to say what had been known and believed for a long time better than it had ever been said before. Poets like Dryden, Pope, Swift, Johnson, and Goldsmith all belong to the Augustan period. Its poetry is very different from the poetry of the Romantic movement half a century later with Wordsworth, Byron, Keats, Shelley, and so on, where there was very much an emphasis on the telling of personal experience.

George Crabbe, who we are going to consider now, was strange in that, although he overlapped both movements in time, he was outside the Augustan school and was really also outside the Romantic school. He didn't fit into either. Could we read his extract from *The Village* now.

> Anon, a figure enters, quaintly neat,
> All pride and business, bustle and conceit;
> With looks unalter'd by the scenes of woe
> With speed that, entering, speaks his haste to go, . . .
> A potent Quack, long versed in human ills
> Who first insults the victim whom he kills;
> Whose murd'rous hand a drowsy Bench protect,
> And whose most tender mercy is neglect.
> Paid by the Parish for his attendance here,

He wears contempt upon his sapient sneer;
In haste he seeks the bed where Misery lies
Impatience mark'd in his averted eyes;
And, some habitual queries hurried o'er
Without reply he rushes on the door.[7]

[*During the reading of this poem, there was much laughter.*]

Dave: God, what a line! 'Whose most tender mercy is neglect.'

Chairman: There was a lot of laughter while you were reading this passage, but this is a portrait of a doctor.

Hilary: This just doesn't touch on the concept of how medicine should be practised now.

Rod: It's almost like the performance of a locum service. 'As he rushes in the door he's already writing out the bill.'

Chairman: Is it so extreme as to be a caricature with no modern relevance?

Gillian: I think it's definitely a caricature, but I also think equally definitely that it has modern relevance. Just because the poem shows an extreme portrait doesn't mean we can't apply it to modern days. Isn't that what a caricature is—an extreme portrait?

David: I don't think this is necessarily a caricature, I think this could be a portrait of some present-day doctors—but not many.

Chairman: Are there any lines which are specifically relevant to the present day?

David: 'With speed that, entering, speaks his haste to go'.

Brendan: The third line is really excellent—'With looks unalter'd by the scenes of woe'.

Hilary: I think the second-last line, 'And, some habitual queries o'er'. He seems to be going through the routine just as quickly as he can.

Doug: And the fourth-last line supports that: 'In haste he seeks the bed where Misery lies'.

Rod: I think the sixth line, 'Who first insults the victim whom he kills', has got a message. You often hear doctors bawling patients out for not looking after themselves, or not taking their tablets.

Chairman: Let's have a look at something lighter now, two paragraphs from different sections of a relatively modern novel, A. J. Cronin's *The Citadel.* Cronin, as you know, is a doctor.

'I came down here full of formulae, the things that everybody believes, or pretends to believe. That swollen joints mean rheumatism. That rheumatism means salicylate. You know, the orthodox things! Well I'm finding out that some of them are all wrong. Take medicine, too. It seems to me that some of it does more harm than good. It's the system. A patient comes into the surgery.

He expects his "bottle of medicine". And he gets it, even if it's only burnt sugar, soda carb, and good old aqua. That's why the prescription is written in Latin–so he won't understand it. It isn't right. It isn't scientific. And another thing. It seems to me that too many doctors treat disease empirically, that's to say, they treat the symptoms individually. They don't bother to combine the symptoms in their own mind and puzzle out the diagnosis. They say very quick, because they're usually in a rush, "Ah! headache–try this powder", or "you're anaemic, you must have some iron". Instead of asking themselves what is *causing* the headache or the anaemia–'. He broke off sharply. 'Oh! I'm sorry! I'm boring you!'

* * *

'I usually have a course of injections at this time of year. I'm subject to hay fever. You know all about hay fever, I presume?'

'Yes', he answered. 'What injections do you have?'

She mentioned the name of a well-known preparation.

'My old doctor put me on to that. I have great faith in it'.

'Oh that!' Nettled at her manner, he was on the point of telling her that the faithful remedy of her faithful doctor was worthless, that it had achieved its popularity through skilful advertising on the part of the firm who produced it and the absence of pollen in most English summers. But with an effort he restrained himself. There was a struggle between all that he believed and all he wished to have. He thought defiantly, if I let this chance slip, after all these months, I'm a fool. He said, 'I think I can give you the injection as well as anyone'.

'Very well. And now about your fees. I never paid Dr Sinclair more than one guinea a visit. May I take it that you will continue this arrangement'.

A guinea a visit–it was three times the largest fee he had ever earned! And more important still, it represented his first step into the superior class of practice he had coveted all these months.[8]

Chairman: Is this a good passage?

[*General comment*] Yes.

Chairman: Why?

Brendan: It describes the metamorphosis of a young doctor . . .

Liz: It certainly does!

Brendan: . . . almost the evolution of a young doctor to a Collins Street specialist.

Nicholas: It's also good because, at least in me, it produces a conflict. It seemed to portray the conflict of the good and the bad within an individual. He more or less understood the principles of medical practice and yet eventually descended to an absolutely wrong action despite that realization.

David: What he did in the second paragraph may have been right, but done for the wrong motive. It may not have been bad medicine. If the woman believes so intently in the injection, then it is probably a very good idea to give her the injection. If she comes in wanting this 'useless' preparation, which has kept her hay fever away, and if this is the only satisfaction she has had, then it is probably right to give it.

Chairman: What was his dilemma?

Gillian: I think it shows how his ambition overcame his morals.

Chairman: Gillian, someone once said that whenever one's interests clash with one's ideals, one's interests win out.

Gillian: I agree with that.

Jane: The passage is portraying something which a lot of people say is inevitable in the development of a doctor: that a young person's ideals gradually finish up just like this person in the passage, and that doctors become vulnerable to material gain. To me, this is just revolting. I hope it never happens to me.

Colin: I would agree with Jane in relation to the second part of the passage, but I think the first paragraph has a different message. It says something which is important in the practice of medicine: often there is no point in chasing a diagnosis when you know that it is not going to improve your treatment of the symptoms. If the establishment of a diagnosis is not going to alter the management, then symptomatic treatment is more justified. While one must try and find a diagnosis, you've only got to try up to a point. Once you have reached the point where, even if you do find it, it's of no benefit to the patient, then I think it's right to stop.

Chairman: That's a very valid medical point.

Stuart: Coming back to Jane's point about material gain, I don't think he knew he was going to get a guinea for his consultation before he'd done it.

David: Yes, but he is talking about 'letting his chance slip after all these months'. Presumably he knew she was a pretty high-class sort of patient.

Robert: Yes, it says here 'there was a struggle between all that he believed and all he wished to have.'

Chairman: I think that is the key line.

Rod: There's a second point in this. I don't think this fellow would have made a very good doctor anyway because he likes everything to be scientific and cut and dried. He can't accept the value of placebos. He says it isn't right, it isn't scientific.

Jane: That's what he learnt when he first came out of medical school, but I think that as soon as he started practising he realized that was wrong. He is now saying that these things don't apply.

Chairman: In a way I agree with Jane, there is a feeling of the doctor's maturation through the first paragraph.

Rod: But that doesn't apply in the second paragraph. He says that he *could* tell her it was a worthless medicine, but he doesn't because he wants her as a patient. He doesn't want to frighten her off.

Chairman: That's a long step from the scientific idealism isn't it?

David: In the first paragraph he's saying 'even if it is only burnt sugar, soda carb. and good old aqua'—it isn't right. But in the next paragraph he gives her something which is just as useless. It's a complete contradiction of what he believed in.

Rod: He still thinks it's useless, but he's giving it to her for a different reason.

Chairman: For what reason could he have done this? Could we be a bit more charitable, without necessarily saying we agree with it?

David: He could be hard up.

Gillian: I think you can be completely charitable, because I think he's describing something which will be inevitable. Not necessarily from the point of view of money, but we all have to lose our ideals to a certain extent. We always seem to, and this just seems to be one of them.

Jane: Well I just hope that isn't true.

Gillian: I'm only being realistic.

Rod: You've got to be realistic to be a doctor.

Jane: But you can be idealistic as well as being realistic. They are not incompatible.

Rod: The two don't go together.

[*Many students in the group disagreed.*]

Robert: You can have your ideals, but you must realize what you can actually get done.

Chairman: Gillian, can you see yourself taking the step that he took?

Gillian: No I can't.

Chairman: Can any of you here see yourself taking this step?

Some students: Yes.

Liz: I would have finished up giving this woman the stupid injection.

David: And if you don't give it to her, she'll go out to another doctor and get it from him.

Stuart: Exactly.

Chairman: Well, can you see yourself doing what he did for *his* reason?

Students [*together*]: No.

David: I don't know we can be sure what his reasons were.

Gillian: They were financial.

Chairman: Can you see yourself in that position?

David: Well if I was totally honest with myself I would say 'possibly yes', but I hope not. A doctor now has a guaranteed financial income. A doctor in England then, especially a young doctor, trying to build up a practice, had a pretty stiff time of it. Even so, today we seem to spend 90 per cent of our time in public fighting about money.

Hilary: I was just wondering how much time had elapsed between the first paragraph and the second in the life of the doctor.

Chairman: I can't answer that from memory, Hilary, but I think it was a few years.

Let's consider a very short passage now. It's from a short story written by John Brown, who was himself a doctor, and is called 'Rab and His Friends'. Incidentally, you may have noticed how many of today's authors were doctors. Chekhov was a doctor, Somerset Maugham, John Brown, George Crabbe, and A. J. Cronin were all doctors.

> [Medical students] . . . get over their professional horrors, and into their proper work; and in them pity as an emotion, ending in itself or at the best in tears and a long drawn breath, lessens,—while pity as a motive, is quickened and gains power and purpose.[9]

Chairman: What do you think is being said here and what's the truth of it?

Colin: I think what he's saying here is that as you mature, your emotions become more purposeful in helping other people. You don't get involved yourself, but rather try to extract what useful information you can from the patient and use your emotional content to be compassionate. It's not the same compassion you might feel for a normal person or friend.

Chairman: That's a good summary of it. Is this a real medical dilemma?

David: I think it is. If you get emotionally involved with every patient and take home all the worries of every patient you treat, you're either going to finish up worn out or worse. It's not fair on the people outside. If a doctor brings these things home his family suffers. The passage says you try and do the best you can while you're there, but when you're gone you've done your best and try and be satisfied. And it is not always easy to do that. If you get upset about a patient it may not be helpful. For example you might go home thinking about the 42-year-old woman with two children, and what is going to happen to them because there's something wrong with the husband.

Brendan: It seems to be more a matter of being able to partition your emotions. I think that's what he's asking us to do. For example, if you're dealing with one patient and are concerned about him, when you move on to the next patient you have to be able to partition away that involvement with the preceding patient. That's one dilemma doctors have to come to grips with.

Nicholas: He's expressing the ideal situation where you are still very much at one with your patient. You are not sitting down crying about the patient, but you are directing yourself to doing something. The only other comment I would like to make is that that's not always what really happens. It's rather that the pity and emotion tend to go altogether, and *no* feeling is more of a problem than emotional involvement.

Doug: I think loss of feeling is a thing that we all feel happening to us. I don't think you can get by as a medical student without it happening, especially if you are going to see a large number of patients.

Chairman: He is drawing a distinction in this passage between the sort of emotional involvement which is tearful and undermining and impotent, and the emotional involvement which is concentrated and focused into something which is going to be used purposefully, perhaps to alleviate suffering or to increase the efficiency of your medical care. He certainly is not arguing for an elimination of the emotional element in patient care. Would any of us be arguing for that?

Students: No.

Colin: I think the argument for this emotional involvement is highlighted by first-year residents when they first get the responsibility of looking after a patient. A lot of residents seem to go back from the second sort of pity to the first ineffective type.

Chairman: Let's take this discussion a little further with a consideration of the last literary passage for today. This comes from Thomas Mann's novel *The Magic Mountain*, a book which won the Nobel Prize for Literature in 1929. The magic mountain is a tuberculosis sanitorium. The patients who are there for care reflect on many aspects of life. In the novel there is this passage relevant to our present discussion.

> He had settled down as one of the physicians who are companions in suffering to the patients in their care; who do not stand above disease, fighting her in the armour of personal security but who themselves bear her mark–an odd, but by no means isolated case, and one which has its good as well as its bad side. Sympathy between doctor and patient is surely desirable, and a case might be made out for the view that only he who suffers can be the guide and healer of the suffering. And yet–can true spiritual mastery over a power be won by him who is counted amongst her slaves? Can he free others who himself is not free? The ailing physician remains a paradox to the average mind, a questionable phenomenon. May not his scientific knowledge tend to be clouded and confused by his

> own participation rather than enriched and morally reinforced? He cannot face disease in clear-eyed hostility to her; he is a prejudiced party, his position is equivocal.[10]

Liz: The first part of the passage seems to be saying that you can't be a good doctor without having experienced sickness.

Gillian: He dices that after a while.

Dave: There's a paradox right in the middle of it.

Rod: I think maybe he feels the best doctor is the doctor who has experienced illness and then got over it. In a way he then embodies the experience of having been ill.

Nicholas: I think he's arguing against that. He's saying . . .

Chairman: How has he achieved the technique of his argument in this passage?

Robert: The phrase 'And yet' is central.

Gillian: And that is followed by a lot of questions to which he gives his own answers.

Chairman: This is not an easy passage. He changes his emphasis through the paragraph. We start off by talking about a *compassionate* physician and halfway through we are talking about an *ailing* physician. It's a clever but slightly sneaky change. He pretends to be weighing up the two sides, while all the time he is putting forward a definite opinion.

Rod: Aren't the first few lines talking about an ailing physician? Physicians who are 'companions in suffering' and who 'do not stand above disease'?

Gillian: No, I don't think he's talking literally there. He's referring to a doctor's compassion for the people who have an illness, rather than the physician actually experiencing it. I think it means the effort of understanding what the patient is suffering without actually suffering it yourself as a doctor.

Hilary: I think it does sound like the doctor himself is suffering from the same condition as the patient.

Brendan: No, it says they do not 'stand above disease'. He's expressing a companionship with the patients who are suffering.

Chairman: I think he is referring to what Gillian and Brendan say, because the passage claims that this companionship with one who is suffering has both its good side and its bad side.

Rod: Doesn't it say that he bears the mark of disease himself?

Gillian: Yes, but it is only the mark of disease because he understands what the patient is experiencing.

Chairman: Well, here we have two opinions again. We have Brendan and Gillian who believe the experience of sickness is being used metaphorically and Rod and Hilary who believe that it is being used literally.

Robert: And I say that I don't think it matters all that much which the author is meaning–to the message of the passage.
David: Yes, the author is recommending the detached position.
Chairman: This has been a very long session. I'm very tired and I am sure you are too.
Gillian: I'm pooped!
Chairman: Thank you again for your concentration and efforts.

ESSAY 3

THE DEMANDS OF DOCTORSHIP

There is a limit to human sympathy.

It is difficult to answer the eternal question of how a human being can achieve happiness. Philosophers have been discussing it for centuries. Some say it is realized by ordering one's life according to God's law, or to a moral law which one perceives intuitively, or to behaviour which the majority opinion holds as 'virtue'. Others have claimed that happiness is found in living a 'natural' life, or in the search for knowledge, or in helping our fellows. And still others place the pursuit of self-realization, self-knowledge or self-gratification ahead of all. The many alternatives would seem to exclude a simple answer.

As the professional performance of a doctor or a nurse is dependent, to some extent, on his or her sense of inner happiness and harmony, I think this question is worth considering further. My own view is this. It seems to me that we cannot be happy unless our life has three things. First, we must have a *sense of self*, a sense of who we are, our merits, and our talents. It does not matter whether this assessment of our personal worth is grand or humble, provided it is the honest admission of what we feel to be true. I think the philosophers have duped us with a supposed difficulty of answering the questions 'Who am I?' and 'What am I?' I believe that if each of us goes to a quiet place and asks these questions of ourselves, then the answers which are of personal relevance (not necessarily those of the ultimate reasons for being) will slowly sound themselves. Most of us know intuitively what we are, and most of us have a special sense which tells us what we need to do or be in order to achieve self-realization and happiness. Men seem to have a great talent to realize that sense of self, but I am convinced that women feel their own identities with equal force, and even greater frustration. To ignore your identity, or to deny it, is a folly, for

> There is a tide in the affairs of men,
> Which, taken at the flood, leads on to fortune;
> Omitted, all the voyage of their life
> Is bound in shallows and in miseries.[1]

Thomas Carlyle, the fiery Scot, noted 'the fallacy of that impossible precept *know thyself* till it be translated into this partially possible one: know what thou canst work at'.[2] Now, while I disagree with his order of importance, there is truth in his view. For it seems to me that the second ingredient of happiness is that our primary awareness of our personal worth should find its expression in our work. Ideally this should be the activity which occupies us most of our time. As doctors and nurses it is obvious that our medical performance will be undermined if we are unhappy in our work. If someone is at war with his work, if he feels confined, frustrated, or unfulfilled, he cannot be happy. Browning once wrote:

> . . . the whole seems to fall into shape,
> As if I saw alike my work and self,
> And all that I was born to be and do,
> A twilight-piece.[3]

Without an awareness of 'all that we are born to be and do' we cannot be happy. I am not saying that achievement of one's ambitions is necessary for happiness—for our ambitions always seem to exceed our capacities: 'Ah, but a man's reach should exceed his grasp, / Or what's a heaven for?'

My third prerequisite for happiness is that our sense of self and our sense of vocational commitment should be reciprocally understood and treasured by the person with whom we share our most private thoughts and emotions: the one for whom we have a spirit of total concern—the one we love. A doctor must have the sympathy and understanding of wife or husband or companion, and particularly tolerance of the time medicine demands. Many doctors take other members of the medical profession for their partners. There is some small advantage in having someone who understands just how demanding medicine can be. The problem of an emergency call which clashes with your five-year-old son's birthday party is unanswerable.

Doctors and nurses, then, are first human beings and must share the joys and burdens of the human family. There are so many paradoxes and ambiguities which are involved in being a member of the human race. Shakespeare called them 'the confounding contraries', and Blake 'the division in the soul of man'. Some of us seem ever torn by the self-contradictory dilemmas of the human state. Think of them: an increase in knowledge brings an awareness of ignorance; solitude leads to loneliness; communality destroys privacy; the greatest commitment produces the greatest vulnerability; man's moral capacity always exceeds his moral ideal; excursions in the imagination frequently exceed the reality; a task achieved is reduced by that achievement; we wish for the unattainable and disregard the available; and however much we achieve there is always a feeling of something more, a feeling of incompleteness. 'And thus we half men struggle'. These are paradoxes which affect both the medical staff and patients alike.

Perhaps the only expression compatible with an understanding of the state of man is a wry smile. But I agree with Coleridge when he said that whereas any man who has thought about the plight of the human condition should be pessimistic, the only spirit compatible with the dignity of man is optimism. So many of our patients are unhappy and in many cases their sadness is related to some aspect of the paradoxes which affect all members of the human family. The same is true of many medical students, doctors, and nurses.

I mentioned before that the loved ones of doctors need to be very patient and understanding of the demands on time made by the practice of medicine. Time is important in another way. In some cases a career decision for medicine anticipates a great amputation of individual potential. For some–particularly those with exceptional or diverse talents–a contract with a medical vocation can impose a severe form of personal atrophy. Medicine is a mistress jealous of time and rarely permits pursuits which are not subservient to her demands. Such individuals can be left with the unhappy dilemma of deciding which of their many talents they must follow.

And what are the actual demands of medical practice? If it is true that human duty has no limits to its extent, yet human capacity has, then the demands of doctorship must come close to that threshold. It seems reasonable to ask if there are certain qualities desirable in a doctor–such as sensitivity, emotional gentleness, and even shyness–which are incompatible with the emotional, psychological, and bodily demands of medical practice. It has taken me many years to find a literary portrait which sympathizes with the problem of a doctor who is shy:

> 'It's no joke in general practice.'
>
> 'Well, you hear men talk about it as though it were, but I tell you it's much nearer tragedy. Take some poor, raw, young fellow who has just put up his plate in a strange town. He has found it a trial all his life, perhaps, to talk to a woman about lawn tennis and church services. When a young man *is* shy he is shyer than any girl. Then down comes an anxious mother and consults him upon the most intimate family matters. 'I shall never go to that doctor again,' says she afterwards. 'His manner is so stiff and unsympathetic.' Unsympathetic! Why, the poor lad was struck dumb and paralysed. I have known general practitioners who were so shy that they could not bring themselves to ask the way in the street. Fancy what sensitive men like that must endure before they get broken in to medical practice. And then they know that if they do not keep a face of stone, their patient will be covered with confusion. And so they keep their face of stone, and earn the reputation perhaps of having a heart to correspond.[4]

It is significant to see just how many 'quiet' students respond to this passage in our sessions.

There is an effect produced by the actual practice of medicine, which is alien to the best practice of medicine. A vocation can mark a person, and whatever the profession wishes to believe, the public is sensitive to traits in their doctors which have been left by the trials of practice. For some doctors and nurses, the ideal they wish for exceeds their capacity and gradually becomes lost. For them, the undulating line of feeling, sentiment, and compassion, gradually becomes straightened. For them, the importance of passive listening becomes engulfed by their active capacities: they become doers rather than receptors. The unceasing demands of doctorship cause them to become forceful, speaking with that tone of exaggerated authority which betrays insecurity.

Doctors and nurses work under conditions of sustained responsibility and stress. A man or woman can only endure a certain amount of emotional and physical adversity. What is beyond that either annihilates us, or passes us by and leaves us apathetic. For a few, this is the outcome of a selfless commitment. But most of us like to feel we illustrate the view that 'the soul's specific gravity constantly reasserts itself as less than that of the sea of troubles into which it has been thrown'. Are we, as students and doctors, aware of the price we pay for our bouyancy? Does medical practice bring changes creeping on us–slow and unrecognized changes, which arise for our protection but which are detrimental to the most delicate and vulnerable qualities of doctorship? One of America's finest writers, Nathaniel Hawthorne, captured some of these subtle qualities in this passage from his mysterious novel, *The Scarlet Letter:*

> A man burdened with a secret should especially avoid the intimacy of his physician. If the latter possesses native sagacity, and a nameless something more–let us call it intuition; if he shows no intrusive egotism, nor disagreeably prominent characteristics of his own; if he has the power, which must be born with him, to bring his mind into such affinity with his patients that this last shall unawares have spoken what he imagines himself only to have thought; if such revelations be received without tumult, and acknowledged not so often by an uttered sympathy as by silence, an inarticulate breath, and here and there a word, to indicate that all is understood; if to these qualifications of a confidant he joined the advantages afforded by his recognised character as a physician–then, at some inevitable moment will the soul of the sufferer be dissolved and flow forth in a dark but transparent stream, bringing all its mysteries into the daylight.[5]

The majority of us are not 'born with' such qualities, so we might ask at what cost, and with what violence to the rest of our personality, do we achieve them? Can we spread ourselves so widely that our effectiveness is reduced? George Crabbe, the eighteenth-century doctor, poet, and preacher, wrote some poignant lines on just this problem:

> Circles in water, as wider they flow,
> The less conspicuous in their progress grow:
> And when at last they touch upon the shore
> Distinction ceases, and they're viewed no more.
>
> His love, like that last circle, all embraced,
> But with effect that never would be traced.[6]

There is a problem which faces all doctors and medical students. Unless we strive to maintain the tender talents of health care, we are at risk of taking the first step towards the hideous portrait of a doctor drawn by Crabbe in his poem *The Village*—which we considered in the last session. If we are successful, however, we may reach the twilight of our career with our humanity intact:

> His mere presence leaves the patient with more hopefulness and vitality. The sight of disease affects him as dust does the careful housewife. It makes him angry and impatient. 'Tut, tut, this will never do!' he cries, as he takes over a new case. He could shoo death out of the room as though he were an intrusive hen. But when the intruder refuses to be dislodged, when the blood moves more slowly and the eyes grow dimmer, then it is that Dr Winter is of more avail than all the drugs in his surgery. Dying folk cling to his hand as if the presence of his bulk and vigour gives them more courage to face the change; and that kindly, wind-beaten face has been the last earthly impression which many a sufferer has carried into the unknown.[7]

Do the medical or nursing student selection boards acknowledge the problem of the emotional, intellectual, and psychological reserves required for good medical practice? Are they discussed during the medical school years?

The demands on doctors, students, and nurses are getting greater. Society's concept of what is a 'disease' has been expanded to include many things which earlier ages would not have acknowledged publicly. It embraces conditions which would once have been regarded as the responsibility of the individual to overcome himself, or would have been thought of as social impropriety or overt criminality. One effect of the rise of the social sciences, of the welfare state, and of increased patient expectation regarding health care (together with the decline of the church) is that the health profession is being asked to give help to an ever-widening spectrum of social ills. Loneliness, personal inadequacy, anxiety, addiction, 'deviation', criminality, and patient irresponsibility, are all frequent visitors in the clinic or ward.

We need to ask, is society's expectation incompatible with the profession's capacity? Are the demands of doctorship now beyond the capacity of the average doctor? What warnings are given to medical students during their training? Are the contractions which are taking place in patient care a consequence of practice rather than a primary professional default? Are modern living and its problems chewing the juice out of the doctor-patient relationship?

SESSION 4

THE ETHICAL LANDSCAPE

Chairman: Today's topic is called The Ethical Landscape. Could we start by answering the question, what are the meanings of the word 'ethics'?

Rod: Professional morals.

Colin: A system of values for the profession to which its members can relate and see whether or not their actions are right or wrong–and to see whether or not their actions are acceptable to other members of the profession.

Chairman: Now do both of those ideas presume obedience to a code of rules?

Rod: No. Not an outside code of rules. Whether or not your morals are decided by yourself or someone outside is a separate issue. What I am saying is that it's adherence to some code of morals.

Colin: But in case of *professional* ethics, it's not really your morals, it's somebody else's–the profession as a whole.

Chairman: That's in the professional context. But I have asked the general question, what does ethics mean? Ethics surely has some meaning other than just the strictly professional one. What are they?

[*Silence.*]

Chairman: It would seem to me from the definitions you have given that ethics is easy: one just obeys the code. One has a set of rules and follows them, and that's that. Now, is ethics always that easy?

Brendan: No; it isn't. Ethics is the application of morals to a course of action. Those morals may not be a clearly defined thing.

David: It's not something you can write down in a tidy way.

Brendan: Well you can write down a code of ethics.

Chairman: Is that the essence of it–the code? I mean, is that the essence of the ethical exercise, the writing down of the code?

Brendan: No, I think it's a set of principles which can be interpreted in various ways. It sets out the general idea.

Chairman: I don't disagree with anything that's been said, I just want an additional dimension of the ethical exercise. [*Silence.*] There is an anecdote told of a philosopher, I think it was Jean-Paul Sartre when he was Professor of Philosophy, which highlights another dimension of the term 'ethics'. A student knocked on Sartre's door and said he had a problem and wanted help. The student said that he had a sick mother and felt an absolute moral duty to look after her as he was the only one available to do it. He also felt that he wanted to fight in the French underground against the Germans. He saw these two things as absolute equals. This highlights the fact that the essence of an ethical or moral exercise is an individual's choice between two things which seem either equally good or equally bad. Ethics implies conflict.

The general point that I am trying to bring out is that anyone can choose between good and bad. The true ethical dilemma comes when the choice is being made between two things which seem equally good or equally bad. Now today I'd like us to explore how one handles that situation, particularly in the medical context.

Dave: That's a good example.

Chairman: As you know, this course is pretty unstructured, but today I would like to try and keep our discussions within a frame of common understanding in relation to what we mean by the term 'ethics'. You have given me one half of the definition, and I have tried to give you another aspect of the concept. With both of these we should be able to loosely frame today's session. There are three short statements which I would like you to keep in the back of your mind so that you are clear about what I mean when I use the word 'ethics'.

1. Ethics is a study of the way we react to moral uncertainty or moral dilemma.
2. A study of ethics attempts to provide a rational framework for understanding the complexities of moral judgment.
3. Such a study is not necessarily concerned with providing any form of specific moral guidance, such as rules of correct behaviour or lists of virtues and vices, and it is not simply a code of professional conduct and manners.

Colin: You're using 'ethics' more as an adjective or as a process rather than as a noun or a thing which can be defined.

Chairman: Exactly Colin. How do we handle the situation where one person, with a fixed moral code and opinion, is in dispute with another person, who, according to his moral codes and beliefs, has another opinion? That could be the situation between two doctors, between a doctor and a politician, or, more importantly, between the doctor and the patient, or the doctor and the relatives. It may even occur between two different relatives in the same family.

Let's consider C. P. Snow's novel, *The Masters*, and in particular three short paragraphs in three successive chapters. They are all relevant to the theme, 'Should a man who is dying be told that he's dying?' In this case the man is the master of a university college–Lady Muriel is his wife, and Joan his daughter.

'He went into hospital last night. They put a tube down him this morning and sent him home. The results came through just before dinner. It is utterly hopeless. At the very most–they give him six months.'

'What is it?'

'Cancer. Absolutely inoperable! . . .'

'Yes, we've heard his sentence,' said Jago. 'But there is one last thing which seems to me more ghastly than the rest. For there is someone who has not heard it.' He paused. Then he said: 'That is the man himself. They are not going to tell him yet.' . . .

'For some reason that seems utterly inhuman,' said Jago, 'these doctors have not told him. He's been given to understand that in two or three months he will be perfectly well. When any of us see him, we are not to let him know any different.'

* * *

'I hope you've already been told that my husband does not realize the true position. He believes that the doctors have overhauled him and found him pretty sound. He has been told that he has the trace of an ulcer, and he believes he will soon be well. I ask you to think before every word, so that you leave him with the same conviction . . . You will understand that I am already acting as I ask you to act. It is not easy for me.'

There was grandeur in her ramrod back. She did not give an inch.

'I am positive,' she said, 'that we are doing right. It is the last comfort we can give him. He can have a month or two in peace.'

'I completely disagree,' Joan cried. 'Do you think comfort is all he wants? Do you think he would take comfort at that price?'

'My dear Joan, I have listened to your views–'

'Then for God's sake don't go on with this farce.' The girl was torn with feeling, the cry welled out of her. 'Give him his dignity back.'

* * *

'He's quite certain he'll soon be well,' Jago said, 'that is the most appalling thing'.

'You would have told him?'

'Without the shadow of a doubt.'

'I'm surprised that you're so convinced,' said Winslow, ready to disagree.

'I'm utterly convinced.'

'I don't like to suggest it, but I'm inclined to think that Dr Jago may be wrong.' Winslow glanced round the table. 'If I'd had to

> make Lady Muriel's decision, I think I might have done the same. I should have thought: this will mean for him a few days or weeks of happiness. It's the last happiness he'll get—he ought to have it if it's in my power. Do any of you share my view?' . . .
>
> 'No,' said Jago. 'You're presuming where no one has a right to presume.' His tone was deep and simple, no trace of awkwardness left. 'There are a few things no one should dare to decide for another man. There are not many serious things in a man's life—but one of them is how he shall meet his death'.[1]

Chairman: Who would like to start?

Nicholas: This is a passage which brings up the great question of whether or not to tell the patient about his fatal illness. That's the crux of it. We are dealing here with a particular situation, and because these decisions are all case-related you can't have a blanket answer for it. You have to consider the particular context and the character of the patient before you decide whether what's happening is good or bad.

Chairman: Good. A number of things have been said and done by a large number of people in this passage, would you like to comment on any of them?

Nicholas: Yes, I was particularly struck by the last paragraph, Jago is speaking: ' "You're presuming where no one has a right to presume." His tone was deep and simple, no trace of awkwardness left. "There are a few things no one should dare to decide for another man. There are not many serious things in a man's life—but one of them is how he shall meet his death".' One of the things which is particularly striking about that paragraph is that doctors do exactly that: they *do* decide how a man should meet his death. They tend to take a patient's life in their hands. They do it not only in this context but in all sorts of ways.

Chairman: You say some doctors do, but what have the doctors done in this passage?

David: They have told him he's going to get better which is absolutely untrue.

Rod: I don't think they've done exactly that. They have told the wife—in a way they have left the decision up to her.

David: But they *have* suggested to the patient that he is going to be well.

Chairman: Well, David said the doctors have lied and Rod says they haven't. Let's just have a look at what's said. ' "For some reason that seems utterly inhuman," said Jago, "these doctors have not told him. He's been given to understand that in two or three months he will be perfectly well." ' Then, later on, Lady Muriel says, ' "He believes that the doctors have overhauled him and found him pretty sound. He has been told that he has the trace of an ulcer, and he believes he will soon be well." '

Rod: I'm not saying that they haven't actually lied to the patient, I'm saying that maybe it wasn't the doctors who made the decision not to tell him.

Liz: Yes, if I was making Lady Muriel's decision I'm not sure I wouldn't have done the same.

Rod: That's my point, perhaps it's Lady Muriel who has made the decision not to tell him, not the doctors. But I suppose you could argue the other way and say that the doctors have also made the decision not to tell him if Lady Muriel asked them not to.

Nicholas: In that case they would have told Lady Muriel first, so they've already embarked on the active path of going around the patient.

Gillian: That's true; it's much easier for doctors if they skirt around the decision like that. That's why they sometimes pass the responsibility off on to the wife.

David: What right have the doctors got to ask *her* what she thinks? Why should *she* be asked, 'Do you want us to tell your husband or not?'

Rod: She might know how he'd take it . . .

David [*raising his voice*]: I think the patient has the right to be told straight away.

Many students [*trying to speak together*].

Colin: I think it's very much like Nick says, you can't generalize, Jago is trying to generalize the situation. In the last four lines he is suggesting that everyone should be told as though this was some sort of absolute truth, or absolute recommendation. On the other hand, Winslow's approach is deficient in human understanding. I don't think he shows enough understanding of the case to comment the way he has.

Gillian: I think the doctors are shirking their responsibility. They're telling the patient what he wants to hear.

Chairman: That's a presumption.

Gillian: O.K., well what they *think* the patient wants them to say.

David: Obviously the patient wants to hear that he's going to get better. He also wants that to be true.

Gillian: I agree with that, the patient would want to hear the truth.

Chairman: The doctors have done two things. First, they haven't told him, and second, they have given him to understand that in two or three months he will be perfectly well. Now are these two things different? Can the doctors' course of action be justified under any circumstances? Colin said it would vary with the circumstances, but would it?

Rod: Yes.

Hilary: I think you can justify omitting truth in certain rare circumstances. But I don't think you could ever justify an outright lie.

Gillian: I don't think there's any difference. Omitting the truth in any situation and knowing that you are doing it to create the exact opposite of the truth, is the same as telling a direct lie!

Rod: Yes; it's exactly the same thing! What do you say? You don't say, 'You've got a cancer', so you let the guy think he's going to get better.

Liz: But you don't have to commit yourself, you can say, 'I'm not sure.' You can be noncommital.

Robert: Being wishy-washy?

Liz: It's not being wishy-washy! You can say you've 'found a tumour', or, 'something's there', without actually saying it's cancer.

Jane: I don't think you could really ever justify not telling a patient the truth or telling a direct lie, certainly not telling them the opposite of the truth. A person's death is really a very personal thing.

Chairman: Well Gillian has said there's no difference between not telling the patient the complete truth of the clinical situation, and telling a patient who's going to die that in two or three months he will be *perfectly well.* Now it seems to me that there are two different things being discussed. Can we envisage any circumstances where either of them would be the correct thing to do?

David: I think there *is* a difference between them. I would never be prepared to tell a patient they were going to get better if they weren't. I couldn't have that on my conscience. But I would be prepared to withhold information in a very unusual circumstance. In most cases I would want to tell them. It strikes me that as soon as you don't tell the patient the truth you come up against all of these problems where people say, 'Which of us has told him what?', or 'Are we going to react?', and 'Where are we going to be evasive?'—all of these problems start to creep in. The simplest thing and the most sensible thing would be to tell them the truth.

Liz: And you also get the problem that if you are wishy-washy about it, some patients will become suspicious. Then they'll start to get scared and have fears because they feel that you're not telling them the truth. Those patients are really left up in the air.

Stuart: I think it's fair to err on the side of optimism in the common clinical situation where you don't know what the prognosis is going to be. Many clinical circumstances are liable to professional error; some patients who come in and who are told they only have a few months to live, can live on happily for a number of years. I think in that case omission could be slightly justified—where you can't be 100-per-cent positive of the clinical outcome.

Gillian: That's a different point.

Brendan: That's not what we are discussing.

Chairman: It is a different point, but I think it's a valid one.

Brendan: There is another point: you can tell a patient the truth and yet leave them with some hope. You can tell a patient what is basically truthful and say to them the chances are 'such and such . . . and so and so.' 'You could be gone in a year, but there are cases who have lived longer.' If you give certain people all the information, they will pick and choose what they want to hear out of what you've said, and they will believe what they'd like to believe out of what you've said. They adjust according to their own needs. You don't really have to tell them what they want to know, just give them all the information and they'll sort it out themselves. If a patient wants to believe that they are going to be the 1 per cent that does have a remission, then they are going to believe it. If on the other hand they want to adjust to dying, then they'll adjust.

Hilary: I would like to question the concept of making a quote on the time that a patient is going to live. I'd like to question the approach of saying it's six months or a year that you have to live, or something like that. I think it's wiser to give them just some general idea of the possibility of the outcome and not to put a time limit on it because people cling to something like that.

Gillian: But don't they often ask you for a time? Frequently they say, 'How long will it be?'

Hilary: You shouldn't answer that!

David: Yes, I think then the doctor should be as vague as possible.

Gillian: But what if they keep asking?

Robert: If you don't know, you don't know! You can't just make up a prognosis.

Nicholas: It's often said that you shouldn't quote statistics at a patient. But what about just quoting survival statistics to a patient when they ask 'How long doctor?'

Robert: That's fine, but it's quite different from saying straight out 'You've got six months!' Using Nicholas's approach you can say indirectly that they've got a reasonable chance or otherwise.

Liz: No; I wouldn't like to do that.

Nicholas: I'm not so sure. I think if I was in a situation like that I would want to have some idea of the chances. But you wouldn't present it in a statistical framework to the patient. You wouldn't tell them that 10 per cent of patients are going to be dead in such and such a time.

Robert: No, you wouldn't be that specific, you wouldn't put it in a cold-hearted way.

Stuart: I read the other day that someone who had a 30 per cent chance of survival was told by the doctor that he had a one in three chance of making it. I think that's not a bad way of saying it, because it's a true indication, yet it also allows for the possibility that they might die in the near future.

David: It does come back to the fact that different sorts of patients are going to accept different sorts of presentation of their prognosis. It really does depend on the circumstances.

Chairman: We opened this session by trying to decide if there was a possibility of finding rules which could guide us in this particular ethical area. From what you have said so far on this issue it would seem this is a very complex equation.

Rod: One of the things which is important is to decide whether it's more important for the patient to have a happy life or a happy death.

Gillian: Why do *you* have to choose?

Rod: Well, an incurable patient might live happily for six months and die just like that [*snapping his fingers*] in a car accident. Not telling him would have saved him unhappiness.

Gillian: Yet, but this man is not going to die like that. Lady Muriel is saying that she's not telling him because he may have a happier life for a bit longer. But he's dying of cancer.

Brendan: Nearly all patients know they are dying!

Robert: Rubbish!

Brendan: Well they've got a pretty good idea. If a whole lot of people in the hospital come and feel their liver, and then the doctor sends them off for two liver scans and a whole lot of strange tests, they all know!

Rod [*interrupting*]*:* Well if they all know, why bother telling them! There's not a problem.

Six students [*all angrily trying to speak together*].

Brendan: It's better to know than always to be guessing and not being given the opportunity to adjust properly.

Rod: What about a woman who comes in for an examination of a simple condition and the doctors find something during the investigation which was unexpected and is serious? Now the serious condition wasn't affecting her life at all at this stage. Are you justified in messing up the patient's life by telling them that they have something that's serious even though it isn't affecting them? Wouldn't it be better to let the patient go out and live their life without fearing death all the time? I think it's better that the patient should go out and have four years of happy life, and then one year of fear when the underlying condition becomes clinically obvious.

Stuart: I think the context of what Rod said is perfectly fair. A number of people come into hospital and something is found that is totally unrelated. If they hadn't been told it was there they would have been perfectly happy.

Liz: Yes, but that's an uncommon situation.

Chairman: That example *is* a side issue, but it's an important one and I am glad it has been brought out.

Brendan: It's very rare—normally a patient presents and they've got something wrong, and it's *that* they're worried about, and it's *that* we have to make a decision about telling them. You don't really need a code of ethics, all you need to do is to be sensitive when you approach the patient, and not shy away. They will ask you what they want to know. They'll indicate to you how much they want you to tell them. If you don't run away, then you will handle it.

Chairman: Would you ever offer information when a patient hasn't asked?

Dave: That depends on whether it's a direct 'ask' or a roundabout 'ask'.

Brendan: Yes, I think that can be handled delicately by simply saying to the patient, 'Is there anything more that you want to know?' Put it as a general question.

Chairman: If under those circumstances the patient said nothing, would you then say nothing even though you know the patient has a fatal prognosis?

Rod: I think patients usually don't ask because they're too frightened to ask, so you shouldn't push it onto them.

Chairman: What about when a patient *does* directly ask?

Liz: I think you should tell them.

Colin: I disagree in some situations. We had a patient recently who had emphysema. She knew that her mother had died of emphysema. She came into hospital and she was obviously in the last stages of emphysema with respiratory failure, and pulmonary problems. Now I think everyone knew that she was going to die, but she kept asking the doctor, 'Have I got emphysema? Have I got emphysema?' But she really didn't want to know, because she was scared stiff of it! She was only asking the question to be told that she didn't have it.

Robert: Apparently that is quite a common reaction in patients who are dogmatically asking you a question. They really don't want to know the answer.

Gillian: Could you justify not telling her anything?

Gillian, Rod, Dave, and Robert [*all trying to speak together*].

Nicholas: You're trying to decide what's in the patient's mind.

Robert: I'm not trying to decide anything.

Chairman: I want the group to help me now. I'm not clear at this moment what the group's feelings are about what the doctors did in this passage: ' "He's been given to understand that in two or three months he will be perfectly well." ' Who, around this table, would have done that?

Gillian: No.

Hilary: No.

Jane: No.

Brendan: No.

Male students: No.
Rod: It depends on the circumstances.
David: We've got the circumstances in the passage.
Chairman: Yes; I think we have: it says here ' "Cancer. Absolutely inoperable!" ' They are the medical circumstances. Can you justify offering an optimistic prognosis of 'in two or three months you will be perfectly well' in those circumstances?
Gillian: I don't think there's any justification for that. I don't think there's any justification for making him understand that in two or three months he's going to be well.
Chairman: O.K., Gillian. Well then, now you *do* draw a differentiation between simply not telling a patient the complete clinical picture, and telling him the opposite of the truth.
Gillian [*laughing good-naturedly*]*:* Yes, I do.
Rod: I'm not prepared to say I definitely would, or I definitely wouldn't. I would want to hold my opinion until I considered the specific case in front of me.
Colin: I don't think you can make a decision if you haven't got enough information. You haven't enough information on what this person is like.
Gillian: I don't think it matters.
Chairman: Some people here say that, as a guiding principle in their practice, they would never deceive a patient irrespective of the lack of information. Colin and Rod say they can't make up their minds and would wait. Can either Rod or Colin envisage a situation where they might take the course of action that these doctors took?
Colin: Yes; the lady who Rod just outlined before with a serious disease which has turned up unexpectedly in the course of investigation into another condition, and which is not producing symptoms at the moment.
Chairman: You would actually tell that woman that she is going to be better in two or three months?
Colin: No, I wouldn't tell her she's going to be better.
Chairman: Well that's the point at issue!
Gillian: That's right!
Rod: I know of a patient who came in who had a fever and cancer of the liver, and it turned out the fever was not related to the cancer of the liver, and the fever got better. I think I'd have told her she was going to be perfectly well and let her go home.
Liz: I wouldn't do that.
Gillian: That's stupid, she's going to come back and it would be perfectly obvious that she's not going to be well.
Rod: What's to stop you sitting down and discussing it *then*?
Chairman: One at a time please!
Jane: In a case like that, if somebody came in with a comparatively

mild condition which wasn't really affecting them, and then a carcinoma is discovered, the doctor has then got to decide whether or not to tell them. But that's not the typical situation.

Liz: Well I think that . . .

Rod [*interrupting*]: Look, you can go up to any patient and tell them . . .

Chairman: Liz first please Rod!

Liz [*trying to speak*]: If a patient came in with a mild condition and you fixed that up, and incidentally you discovered something which, though asymptomatic, was very serious, I would not tell the patient, and in that I agree with Colin and Rod, but I wouldn't tell them they are going to be perfectly well.

Brendan: O.K. Well could I ask you, what if someone came in with a pneumonia and underlying it was a cancer of the lung? The pneumonia was cured and they were perfectly well. What then? Would you tell them they have a cancer of the lung?

Liz: Well, if it was an old man, I wouldn't.

Hilary: I think you should tell them. Because even if it is going to cause distress earlier than it normally would, they've got time to adapt. They have the rest of their lives to consider. They have their families to consider, and everyone around them . . .

[*Considerable noise and debate within the group.*]

Hilary [*trying to continue*]: Imagine if you were going to die . . .

Robert: But I *am* going to die! What I am saying is that nobody is really putting a death sentence on another human being, it's there from the moment we're born.

Gillian: I think you're assuming that immediately somebody finds out they've got cancer, they become unhappy. People can accept the fact that they're dying.

Robert: But as soon as you're born, you're dying!

Chairman: Robert, surely the human significance is quite different. I mean, the human significance of me knowing I'm going to die 'at some time' is quite different from me with a wife and four children facing an immediate prognosis of acute leukaemia?

Hilary: That's right! That's why you've got to tell somebody: so they can make plans to look after their relatives and loved ones.

Colin: I think the approach has to be modified by considering the actual disease. If it's an asymptomatic lung cancer, then it's going to become symptomatic at some time. And in the case of lung cancer, very soon, because the natural history is of very quick growth.

Chairman: Let's look at a fresh point. In the passage, David seized on the point that the relatives have been told, and that the patient hasn't. As all of us realize, around the hospital, this is a very common practice. Many students are given the guidance that the relatives must always be told, but the patient, well . . .

Brendan: I think it should be the other way around.

Chairman: How do we feel about this medical habit of ours of always telling the relatives, but not the patient?

Brendan: It might be a practical thing as much as anything else, because usually when the patient comes back from an operation, the relatives are all hovering around and they are there to tell.

Chairman: I don't think that's the common situation Brendan.

Brendan: Then I think it's a way of palming off the responsibility. It's easier.

Rod: It *is* easier for the doctor to tell somebody else than go face to face with the patient.

Gillian: It seems to me to be dumping it all in the relatives' lap.

Nicholas: There could be an important practical reason: you might get a greater insight into how the patient will react. By telling the relatives first you get additional information into the patient's background, and how the patient might react to it. It's really an appendix to your history.

Gillian: But you have to go along and tell the patient as well. You can't just leave it with telling the relatives. You've not done your duty when you have told the relatives.

Brendan: Another aspect is that quite often a doctor is scared witless by going to tell the patient, and they like to have the support of the relatives. If the patient becomes distressed, the relatives who have already been told are there to meaningfully comfort him. I don't think it's easy telling someone they're going to die. You can't just walk away and then just leave them there on their own. I think that if the wife or the relatives and loved ones are just outside the door, and prepared, and come in straight away, it would be a help.

Liz: And don't you think the patient would feel better if he knew that the relatives knew about it.

Gillian: No! I think that the patient should decide whether the relatives should be told or not.

Chairman: Right Gillian, that's another dilemma: that the patient should decide if the relatives are to be told rather than the relatives deciding about the patient.

David: I think that telling the patient, and letting him decide whether or not the relatives should be told, is a lot less ridiculous than speaking to the relatives and asking them should the patient be told. But I think both are probably wrong.

Dave: I don't know what to think at the moment. [*Laughter which Dave ignores.*] I'm just trying to work out what Gillian said about palming off the responsibility. It seems to me that is a very easy way to get out of it, although when you tell someone they are going to die, it's not as though you walk in one day and you give them just a cut and dried statement. I think those who are going to die have a fair idea anyway.

Many students [*speaking together*].

Liz: I don't think many doctors would walk up to a patient and just bluntly say, 'You are going to die.' It's much more subtle than that.

Stuart: Well if they're a moderately intelligent sort of patient, you can start off by telling them, or at least explaining, certain aspects of their disease.

Chairman: In the passage the patient was the master of a university college.

Brendan: If you don't tell him he'll know anyway!

Chairman: You've said that before, and it's an opinion that some of us may disagree with. Saying patients 'always know' is not really helpful, Brendan.

Gillian: Yes, it's just assuming something that may not be right.

Rod: If he's the master of a college he's obviously got some theological background, and I think he would probably get quite a bit of help from above!

[*Laughter.*]

Chairman: Now what about the differing attitudes of Lady Muriel and Joan? Could we read the second paragraph again and refresh ourselves.

> 'I hope you've already been told that my husband does not realize the true position. He believes that the doctors have overhauled him and found him pretty sound. He has been told that he has the trace of an ulcer, and he believes he will soon be well. I ask you to think before every word, so that you leave him the same conviction . . . You will understand that I am already acting as I ask you to act. It is not easy for me.'
>
> There was grandeur in her ramrod back. She did not give an inch. 'I am positive,' she said, 'that we are doing right. It is the last comfort we can give him. He can have a month or two in peace.'
>
> 'I completely disagree,' Joan cried. 'Do you think comfort is all he wants? Do you think he would take comfort at that price?'
>
> 'My dear Joan, I have listened to your views –'
>
> 'Then for God's sake don't go on with this farce.' The girl was torn with feeling, the cry welled out of her. 'Give him his dignity back.'

Nicholas: Lady Muriel has taken the burden of the illness on herself. She's taken it on her own shoulders. She'll be doing the suffering for the dying man.

David: I think she's frightened of how she's going to handle it if he does know. She says to her daughter ' "I have listened to your view—" ' as if to say, 'I'm going to shut my ears to that, I don't want to hear any more of it.'

Gillian: I agree, she's saying, 'I don't want to admit to myself that he's dying, so I am going to kid everyone into pretending that he's not.'

Chairman: Is there anything in the portrait that we're given of her to suggest that she's that sort of person?

David: Yes, 'There was grandeur in her ramrod back.'

Gillian: 'She didn't give an inch.'

Chairman: Nicholas, would you like to come back on that point?

Nicholas: Yes, often a relative feels guilt in this situation, and tends to express this guilt in a last heroic effort on the patient's behalf, which isn't necessarily good, it's just heroic. Because of this woman's strength that was the feeling I got.

Hilary: I think Joan perceives the strain that this artificiality is going to put on the dying man's relationships . . .

Rod: I disagree . . .

Hilary [*continuing*]: But it's a situation that should never arise, I mean I don't think the relatives should be put in the position of pretending. It's a situation which the person who is dying will always detect. He'll realize that there is something wrong with the way they're behaving and he may or may not understand.

Chairman: Lady Muriel does make that point, saying ' "I ask you to think before every word." '

Nicholas: That would be absolutely terrible.

Rod: I would like to disagree with what Hilary said. I don't think Joan is worried about how it's going to affect her relationship with her father . . .

Hilary: No, I didn't say that.

Rod [*continuing*]: It's more that she's concerned about giving him his dignity back. Now Hilary, you're saying she (Joan) is worried about the tension it's going to put on conversations, I don't think you can say she's worrying about that at all . . .

Hilary: But . . .

Rod [*continuing*]: All she wants is for her father to have a respectful death.

Stuart: I think you've misinterpreted what Hilary said.

Hilary: When Joan said, ' "Then for God's sake don't go on with this farce" ', I don't think she's worried about *her* relationship with her father, but she *is* concerned about how her father is going to be affected by this farce.

Chairman: I see. Well Rod, it looks like Hilary's point was a slightly more subtle one than we thought. [*Laughter.*] Rod is saying the fundamental point is that Joan is asking for the father's dignity to be given back, and Hilary is saying that one element of that 'giving the dignity back' would be to avoid creating an artificial farce situation. You are really both saying a similar thing as far as I can see. Do you agree?

Hilary and Rod: Yes.

David: On the other hand you do have some patients who haven't faced any reality during their life, and who don't want to face it now they are facing death. People like that aren't going to admit to themselves their death, even if they do realize it.

Liz: I would like to make a blanket statement. I think everybody should be told what's going to happen to them and then they can make up their mind (as Brendan said before) just what it is they want to believe. If they want to adapt to it they will, if they want to shut it out of their mind, they will.

Chairman: So you would be on the 'Joan' side of the argument?

Liz: Yes.

Gillian: Isn't it true that there is always artificiality even if the relatives have told the patient? After a patient like this has been told, don't the relatives carry on with artificial joviality to try and help him?

Colin: I think that in every family there is more or less a leader, someone who makes the decisions. They accept things and say this is how we are going to cope with them. This passage shows a situation where the leader of the family, the Master, has been nipped off and next in line, the one who's taking up the responsibility of the family, Lady Muriel, is incompetent to do it. She's taking it because she thinks it's her responsibility. Joan, who isn't next in line, really should be doing it.

Nicholas: It really sounds here as if Lady Muriel is the one who's leading the decision-making.

Rod: But that's only because, as Colin said, the husband's gone. He's normally the one who makes all the decisions, but he's not there now so she's doing it.

David: Lady Muriel is the next person in seniority but she is not necessarily the most capable of handling this sort of decision.

Gillian: But the doctors have put her in that position, haven't they?

Chairman: Gillian, the doctors may have put her in that position, but she's an independent human being. She has as much option as Joan to tell or not to tell the husband. Doctors can indicate a line of policy, but each of the relatives, at some stage, is going to make up her own mind as to whether she is going to go along with it. Where does the author want us to side in this Joan–Lady Muriel debate?

Gillian: With Joan.

Robert: With Joan.

Liz: He portrays Joan with a lot more emotion.

Chairman: Would you concede that both Lady Muriel and Joan are working from the premise of what they feel in their heart of hearts is best for their loved one?

Gillian: Yes.

Chairman: Is there any way that these two positions can be resolved? Is there any way that Lady Muriel and Joan will ever agree when they feel what they feel with such intensity?

Hilary: No.

Liz: No.

Jane: No.

Nicholas: I think there could be one; if you brought in a third party, a person who had no interest other than an interest in the welfare of the two people who are in the dilemma. In a situation such as this if there was a third party who had excellent knowledge of the people concerned, he might be able to help.

Chairman: Do you think they could resolve it between themselves as it stands?

Nicholas: I think they have resolved it actually. Lady Muriel has one opinion and Joan has another, but Joan isn't acting on hers, she has agreed to obey her mother. That is a resolution isn't it?

Robert: But it's for one side.

Gillian: Hmm. It's not a resolution in the sense that Joan doesn't agree that she's doing the right thing.

Chairman: Do you see the parallel between this and the example I started the session with, about the student who wanted to do two things but couldn't do both? Joan wants to act for her father's sake, but doesn't want to disobey her mother.

Stuart: Yes.

Jane: I still think you should let the person who is ill decide for themselves.

Colin: Should a doctor go up and ask him, 'Do you want to know if you're dying?'

Jane: No. I am not saying anything like that!

Six students [*trying to speak together*].

Liz: I just want to know what the group's opinion is on something. What do you do, if when you speak to the relatives first (whether or not a clear diagnosis has been made) they say to you, 'Look, I don't want you to tell the patient anything about what's wrong with him.' What do you do then? Do you take it upon yourself to decide that the patient should know and has the right to know, or do you commit yourself to go along with the relatives' request?

Dave: Well I would find out what's wrong with the bloke first then discuss it again with the relatives.

Liz: It was obviously terminal cancer here. But I recently had something to do with a case where even before a diagnosis was made the relatives had asked the doctor not to tell the patient anything.

Chairman: My feeling would be that the relatives' request is just one bit of information which is added to the whole landscape of what's going on, and which forms the background against which you're going to make your decisions as the doctor.

Liz: Would you go against the relatives' request?

Dave: What's all this hang-up about the relatives? It's the *patient* whom the doctor's dealing with.

Liz: The point I'm trying to make is, how responsible is the doctor to the relatives? If they specifically ask you not to tell him, do you have the right to go against what they request?

Chairman: This overlaps with the discussion we had in Session 2, on the relatives' experience of illness. During that session one of you made a point that the closer the patient was to the relative, the more inclination the doctor should have to treat them as one individual and speak to them together explaining things jointly. I thought that was a good point. On the other hand when relatives are much more separate and perhaps not getting on well with the patient a doctor would be less inclined to obey their request.

Gillian: On the other hand you could tell them both separately and let them decide how much they are going to share and relate their knowledge with each other.

Chairman: Would any of you be for a blanket policy of telling all relatives and all patients all of the time?

[*General consensus*] Almost always, but not in every case.

Brendan: As I said before, I think they should all be told because they will believe what they want to believe, and they'll deny what they don't want to believe.

Gillian: I think the whole area of children is a difficult situation because children frequently do ask the doctor what's wrong and that's just so difficult to know what to say.

Chairman: One of the students in another group said she believed we were not open and honest enough with young patients. But I agree with you–it is an exceedingly difficult area.

Could we move on to the next passage now? It is an extract taken from a medical journal on the problem of truth in the clinical context.

> Moral actions can be considered from four points of view; the motivation, the principle, the method or means, and the consequence. To rely exclusively on any single moral parameter can produce all sorts of horrible moral results. For example, if a person subscribed absolutely to the morality of *motivation*, then *any* act could be justified on the basis of 'well, I thought it was for good.' And yet the exclusive adherence to the code of moral *consequence* leads to moral positions which are equally unacceptable. Such a decree would fail to differentiate, say, between two men who had both transmitted the plague to a population, one knowingly and the other in ignorance.[2]

Colin: I think this passage is saying something which we have been saying all along. In morals and ethics there are just so many factors which are involved, that it's very hard when one is faced with making a difficult choice. You have to take so many things in and every element in it has to be counterpoised.

Chairman: So complexity and difficulty is inherent in the ethical equation?

Colin: Yes.

Dave: I think this passage summarizes very well what we've been saying.

Gillian: What it says about the morality of motivation, principle, method and means, and the consequence, is quite helpful.

Colin: I like the way the passage indicates that you really can justify anything if you wanted to by saying you thought it was for good. In the clinical context, that immediately shows up when you're saying, 'Oh I really felt it was best for the person concerned.' By taking that position you may be avoiding the issue. That may be a wrong way of looking at it because you've ignored perhaps what the consequences are.

Nicholas: I think it's ridiculously retrospective, because when you say 'I thought it was for the good' you usually have thought of the consequences and the means. You only find out it was bad after you've actually done it. The passage is helpful in a way: it highlights that there's more than the simple situation in front of you to consider in making an ethical decision. It's obviously arguing against the adherence to a blind principle such as 'I will always tell the patient that they're dying when they are dying'. The passage is asking us to think beyond that, to think of the whole context. What I was saying was that you usually have done that when you say, 'What I was doing I thought I was doing for good.'

Chairman: Are you saying, Nicholas, that if you were convinced that the person who was undertaking a course of action was doing it for a good motive, you'd be more tolerant of their action . . .

Liz: Even if they knew at the time that what they were doing was producing harmful consequences?

Chairman: I agree with Liz's point. You see Nicholas, the acceptance of somebody saying 'I thought I was doing it for good' would lead us to accept somebody like Hitler.

Nicholas: No. I think that in the case of Hitler he would probably argue that his consequences were good as well. According to his moral code, he would feel he was totally justified. The thing is that you wouldn't have a common set of morals with this man. Would you ever try and rationalize morals with somebody like Hitler?

Rod: Well then you can't criticize him if he's got different morals to you.

Nicholas: No, that's not what we're discussing. When you [the chairman] said 'Would you be more tolerant of someone's views if you thought they were working from an honourable motive?', well, that's a funny sort of word 'tolerate'; it doesn't mean accept, it doesn't say it's good, but it does imply that you can understand what he was doing, and why.

Chairman: Nicholas, I understand what you're saying. The point I was making was a separate one: if one does adhere absolutely to the code of the morality of motivation, then, as this passage says, it quickly leads us to absurd moral positions.

Jane: I think people like Nixon and Hitler could equally use this passage to justify what they've been doing. They could say their motivation was right, and their means was right, and the consequence of what they did was right. That's not to say someone outside would agree with what they've done. What I am saying is that they could regard this passage as giving them freedom to do what they did. Provided they were completely alien, morally, from the majority of people, they wouldn't be affected and they would just go ahead.

Chairman: Yes, I see what you mean. I suppose one could argue that there have been times in history when everything that Hitler did was done with some degree of approval from the general populace.

Nicholas [*grimly*]*:* It was in Hitler's case too.

Rod: I think we have misinterpreted this passage if we are looking at it to explain or excuse what people have done. I think it just gives us insight to how we make our moral decisions.

Chairman: I mentioned earlier in the session that 'A study of ethics attempts to provide a rational framework for understanding the complexities of moral judgement.' Is that what this passage does?

Rod: Yes.

Chairman: Now let's have a look at an article which appeared in the newspaper last week which deals with the topic we are discussing.

THE AGE, Tuesday, October 26, 1976

Doctors warned of silence on death

Tell patient or be sued: expert

SYDNEY.–Hospitals and medical staffs could soon face legal action for disclosing or withholding information about a patient's terminal illness without his consent. This is the prediction of Dr. Beverley Raphael, associate professor of psychiatry at the University of Sydney.

Professor Raphael said a patient must be able to exercise his own prerogatives on whether or not he wants this information. 'I can see, in the not too distant future, the situation where a hospital or its medical personnel may be sued for ignoring this sanction, for breaking ethical prohibitions and revealing, without the patient's consent, knowledge concerning him to others,' Professor Raphael said.

'Patients wish to know of their terminal diagnosis in probably 90 per cent of instances. The system's current perception as reflected in doctors is that 90 per cent of patients do not want to know. Surely the system's prerogative is to meet patients' need rather than to impose a view contrary to their needs.'

Professor Raphael said it was common for people, told of a close relative's terminal illness, to decide that the patient is not to be told. In the case of adults it was improper for them to withhold the right to this knowledge from the patient, she said. 'The ideal situation is one in which this knowledge could be received by the family as a whole, supporting and showing their concern for the sick member, so that there are no painful avoidances, or isolating conspiracies of silence,' Professor Raphael said.

Last night a former medical secretary of the Victorian branch of the Australian Medical Association, Dr. A. W. Burton, agreed with Professor Raphael that doctors commonly withheld the information from a patient at the urging of relatives. Dr. Burton is the author of the standard medico-legal text, *Medical Ethics and Law*. He said that doctors normally are guided to act in what they judge to be their patient's best interests. 'It would be a sorry state of affairs if a doctor–acting in the best interests of his patient–has to look over his shoulder to see if what he's doing is in accordance with the law,' Dr. Burton said.[3]

Chairman: What is your response to this newspaper article?

Rod: Anger.

Chairman: Explain, Rod.

Rod: I felt angry with the first half of the article. I think the doctor is the person who should make the decision; the doctor might make a wrong decision, but it's his decision to make.

Nicholas: Jesus!

Jane: Oh no.

Rod: And I don't think there should be people sitting down in the law courts telling doctors that they mustn't do this or that.

Nicholas: Look, that's just terrible. I mean . . . [*pausing*] I mean a doctor isn't God! . . .

Rod [*interrupting*]*:* But neither is the man in the law courts!

Chairman: Let Nicholas speak.

Nicholas: This passage has a lot to say for it because doctors often assume a very authoritarian stance, positions which cannot be justified by any liberal morals or principles. Maybe it is sometimes in the patient's interest, but often it presumes too much. I don't think you can disagree with much of this article.

Rod: I think you can. You can't put a strict rule on things like 'Every patient must be told.' That's far too simplistic.

Nicholas: Well in a way you *can* make it a rule. In a way, just from the premise of justice, you *can* say, 'This should be the case.'

Chairman: Here we have two points of view. Rod is saying that there should not be any rule telling doctors what they must do in relation to what they tell their patients. Nicholas, you're saying the sentiment expressed in the article is that there should be a move back towards the rights of the patient, and this should be encouraged because if the rights of the patient include the right to be told, then they *should* be told.

David: That's good; but the patient might have the *right* to be told without there being *compulsion* on the doctor to tell him. They are two different things.

Rod: I disagree that any such behaviour of doctors should be compulsory.

Chairman: Nicholas, what about the rights of the doctor? What about his or her preferences? Do you see the point: that the doctor has rights just as the patient has rights, and that any dictate forcing the doctor to act in a given way would be against the doctor's rights?

Nicholas: Yes I understand that, and I would answer this way: occasionally the patient's rights infringe on the doctor's rights. But the doctor's decisions will influence the patient to a much greater degree because the patient is not in the same position of power in relation to the doctor. It is the patient who needs protection; it is the patient who is vulnerable.

Rod: In a way it is the doctor who needs protection. If you enforce on a doctor that he must always tell the patients that they have a cancer, you might have doctors actually looking less thoroughly for cancer, less tests will be done for example.

Colin: The argument as presented in the newspaper is very simplistic, and I think it's a pity that it came into a newspaper. It ignores all of the complexities and difficulties in the situation and gives a superficial veneer to the whole thing.

Stuart: It's not a good article.

Jane: I disagree. The point of the article is not just that there should be a law, but that the patient has all of the rights, and that the doctor is really there just to serve the patient. It's really saying that the patient should be completely involved in his own illness, after all, it is *his* illness. And as he should be involved in his own treatment, and his own death, he has the fundamental right to know.

Dave: I agree.

Chairman: So that, inasmuch as the article is reminding doctors of their prime responsibility to the patient, you are for it?

Jane: Yes, and I think that this Dr Burton exhibits the view of a lot of doctors that they have the sole right over the patient on how he's to be treated and what happens to him—have the sole right of his illness. Now that's not justified. Dr Burton is worried about people looking over the doctor's shoulder, well I don't necessarily believe there should be a law, but more importantly, I just don't think the doctor has that sort of right over the patient.

Dave: It strikes me that a lot of doctors see patients as just objects. They don't involve the patient as they should. As Jane said, the patient should be entirely involved with what's going on. After all, it is their illness and it's going to be their death. And this article is reminding us, as you said, of the responsibility that the doctors have to their patients. But I still think that the doctor should be allowed to maintain that little bit of concern for his patient and independence from any absolute law on how he should be behaving. I think he must have the option, if he wishes it, to decide that in a special case, if he thinks it's not in the patient's interest, not to tell them. It may be clinically more responsible for him not to tell the patient what is going on.

Gillian: I want to know if Nick thinks there should be a law. Do you think there should be a law saying that doctors *have* to tell their patients they're going to die?

Nicholas: Well there is a law that says doctors can't kill patients. You agree. Do you object against the law which says that doctors shouldn't kill their patients?

Gillian: I think that's a completely different thing.

Chairman: Nick, Gillian did put a fair question to you.

Nicholas: Well in a way it's similar.

Gillian [*persisting*]: Are you saying 'Yes' or 'No'?

Nicholas [*hesitantly*]: Are we putting . . . I don't want to answer 'Yes' or 'No'—what's the point . . . [*Protests.*] I haven't yet established what sort of law it's going to be, whether it's going to be a principle of medicine such as that in medicine you always work for the good of your patient, or whether it's going to be a law of parliament.

Gillian: I accept that answer but I would like to ask you another question. If the law was an actual law where a doctor could be taken up to court or fined or gaoled for not obeying it . . .

Nicholas: Taken to court for not letting the patient know the full facts about his illness?

Gillian: Yes, do you think that's justified?

Nicholas: Yes, I think it is, because if a patient has decided that the doctor didn't do well by him, that the doctor has made an error, and it's a severe enough situation, then I . . .

Gillian: Don't you think that will influence how a doctor treats his patients–if he knows that if he slips he's got to go to court?

Nicholas: It could. But if a doctor needs the impetus of being taken to court in order to make him tell his patient, then he . . .

Gillian: Don't you think under those circumstances he'll stop thinking about the patient's own good and start thinking about himself?

Nicholas: How do you mean?

Chairman: Say what's in your mind Gillian.

Gillian: Well it's my opinion that there shouldn't be a law because it would influence the doctor's judgement as to whether or not he told, and how he told, the patient. He might really press it, in making sure the patient knows he's going to die, without thinking about *how* he's telling him or what the consequences of telling him will be. The doctor might be in the position of having to rush to make sure he tells him before the patient gets in with legal complaints.

Colin: It might dictate the management without any consideration of the specific patient the doctor is dealing with.

Gillian [*continuing to Nicholas*]: You know how you were saying that the patient should be considered first, well, such a law might act completely against that. I think the doctor might start to think only about himself.

Dave: Yes.

Nicholas: I don't think the law would have to be only that you're going to tell the patient he is to die, but rather that it is quite reasonable to let the patient know exactly what the situation of his illness is.

Hilary: Stating a law like that leaves it wide open for abuse because there is not always a clear-cut situation where the doctor can say, 'You have this or this.' The doctor can't always say clearly, 'You're going to die' . . .

Six students [*trying to speak together*].

Chairman: Please, I ask you again, don't all speak together! Let Hilary finish.

Hilary: Often the doctor can only make a vague statement or discuss it gently with the patient. If he could have himself sued because he didn't clearly tell the patient what was the diagnosis it would be a terrible situation.

Robert: I agree.

David: I think that as far as possible we want to stay clear of having the law courts involved. Nick said before that there was a law which said that doctors shouldn't kill their patients, well I almost think that in certain cases that law should go too.

Nicholas: Wow! You've got terrific judgement.

Chairman: Nick, could I just make a comment to you. The law which says doctors shouldn't kill their patients overlaps with a statutory law that says a doctor can't kill his next-door neighbour, or that one human being can't kill another. But there is no law which really exists which commands an individual to be truthful with the person they are talking to. Do you agree that it's a little different?

Nicholas: But I also think you're over-emphasizing the importance and singularity of the medical profession. I don't think that they are so far removed from the next-door neighbour situation.

Gillian [*to Nicholas*]*:* But do you tell your next-door neighbour how to speak and what to say?

Brendan: The concept of the law invokes the concept of the 'reasonable man'. I think you could easily frame a piece of legislation which wouldn't put anybody in a difficult situation. You could have something which loosely said that the patient mustn't be misled.

Gillian: Well why have it if everyone's already doing that?

Brendan: I agree, I wouldn't want a law. But as a matter of civil rights you could ask why should a doctor be immune from some sort of punishment if he's deliberately misled a patient. Just as he wouldn't be immune from the normal process of torts. Now, every other person in every other job is subject to the law. There can't be a breach of contract in business; you might say that a doctor is in the same position.

Gillian: But I think we mislead people all the time. It's not as though you should be pulled up in court for it.

David: Perhaps the patient ought to have some right of comeback: if he's *grossly* misled by the doctor and if this causes him severe pain and suffering.

Chairman: Well could the Master in the first passage we considered today have grounds for such an action? Would you regard the degree to which he was misled as culpable?

Liz: Yes.

Chairman: Would you regard the doctors in that passage as having a legal case to answer?

David: Are you asking me?

Chairman: Yes.

David: I am almost inclined to think that what was done isn't severe enough for the patient to be able to take a doctor to court.

Nicholas: My God!

Chairman: O.K., you've given your answer!

Rod: I think we're forgetting that the patient's actual treatment does not only involve the treatment of his disease, but it also involves psychological and functional aspects of . . .

Nicholas: Who the hell is the doctor to dictate to the patient . . .

Rod [*shouting*]*:* Well, who the hell else is going to! The guy down in the courts?

Nicholas [*shouting*]: Well why make *any* laws at all?

Rod: Exactly! You're the one that wanted to make the law. Exactly, why make rules at all, that's what I'm trying to say!

Dave: That's right!

Chairman: You've missed Nicholas's point. If you dismiss the courts you undermine the whole concept of 'law'.

Nicholas: Look! The only thing we run on is 'truth' so why not just state it as a principle.

Gillian and Rod [*shouting together*]: You don't need a law!

Chairman: Nicholas, where does your approach leave the concept of professional trust?

Nicholas: How do you mean? [*Pause.*] Well, no, I understand. Professional trust seems to me to be based on candidness. As soon as you start deceiving your patient you're breaching professional trust.

Gillian: But putting a law there isn't going to help it!

Rod: Surely you're questioning professional trust?

Nicholas: If a doctor is prone to breaching his professional trust what comeback does the patient have?

Gillian and Robert: [*trying to speak together*].

Nicholas: Are you saying I don't trust doctors? You're dead right! I don't.

Robert: So you want a law?

Rod: Do you trust lawyers?

Nicholas: No.

Chairman: Can the medical profession survive without the trust of the patients?

[*General agreement*] No, it cannot.

Nicholas: Of course it can't

Chairman: We can say, 'Let's have professional behaviour which will justify that trust', but if we carry that attitude too far and put the profession under too great a scrutiny, then we can chop the legs from under the profession if such scrutiny undermines public confidence in the doctor. Nicholas, do you see the implication of carrying professional criticism too far?

Nicholas: Yes I do, but I would also like to add that while you can't legislate emotion you can legislate to make the doctor responsible. I just want the profession to behave in a certain way. I don't really care whether there is a law or not. I agree completely that it could be destructive.

Chairman: On the other hand Rod, there are defects in the patients' protection against being lied to, as things stand now.

Brendan: It could well be that we don't need a new law. If a patient really knew the law and knew their rights, they could sue a doctor under the existing law.

Chairman: Like Colin, I'm disturbed by this newspaper article, but I may be disturbed for a different reason. I'm disturbed for Nick's reason. That is, why is it necessary for an article like that to appear? Surely we have already gone wrong somewhere if we are receiving this sort of publicity. That is part of what Nick was saying and I agree with it. He was making a further point in relation to the need for a law and I would like us to consider that question in relation to the next passage. It is a further extract from the article 'Truth and Consent', published in the *Medical Journal of Australia.*

> Clinical practice and clinical trials can both involve difficult ethical problems–problems which are not made easier by some external, inflexible, omnipotent legislative dictate telling doctors what they *ought* to do, think and feel. Such rules are alien to the nature of medical practice and ethical judgements, both of which are influenced by the circumstances and opinions of individual patients and doctors. Such decisions should be joint verdicts involving the patient, and family doctor, the specialist, medical administrators, and–when the adult patient so desires–his family. They should consider not only purely medical evidence, but the resources of the family and the patient (economic, emotional, psychological and physical) as well as the ethical issues involved.[4]

Rod: I think this passage highlights the problem of mixing the courts in medical matters. Now let's look at what's happening in America just at the moment. There they have these enormous legal suits against doctors and the whole medical profession is becoming tied down by the fear of legislative recrimination.

Chairman: Could I anticipate Nick's reply and say that this is entirely the medical profession's own fault, that if the doctors had been performing at a better level, this terrible situation in the United States never would have happened. Is that the answer you would have given Nick?

Nicholas: Partly yes and partly no. To some extent I would back up the doctors, but I think doctors may have allowed this situation to arise by deficiencies at the top end. I think this passage does support something I was saying earlier, that such decisions should be joint verdicts involving a lot of people. And the doctor mustn't sit like God.

Dave: I see this passage as saying exactly the opposite of what you are saying, Nick, in that it is arguing against strict legislation.

Nicholas: Just a moment! It does outline what should be done to prevent the need for legislation. In that, I agree with it, for it points the reasons why legislation shouldn't be required if doctors were performing better.

Brendan: I suppose one could say that, when professional trust and responsibility have broken down, as a last resort, the patient should have the option of the law. The law really is only a response to the fact that the patient has been pushed around. If the trust was there all along, you wouldn't need legislation. Basically I believe legislation wouldn't work because you can't tell people the way to behave! That's impractical. But the law *is* always a last recourse for gross negligence.

Many students [*shouting at each other*].

Chairman [*somewhat exasperated*]*:* Come on now, will you speak just one at a time please!

David: This passage says that an ethical decision is not made easier by hanging over the doctor's head some terrible law which says that if you do it wrong, you're in trouble. But I believe that the law should be there for people to take action as a last resort in any case. Perhaps medicine should not be immune from patients who have been grossly wronged having the resort of legal action.

Chairman: I think that's been Nicholas's point all along.

Colin: This passage has an amazing understatement, where it says that 'telling doctors what they *ought* to do, think and feel. Such rules are alien to the nature of medical practice and ethical judgements'. I think that is just so true, but you can't imagine a more self-righteous profession through history than the medical profession.

Rod: The legal profession stands out a lot more.

Stuart: I would like to make a comment on this business of the law, and lawyers. In America, the fundamental difference is that lawyers are permitted to go and solicit clients, and to get a cut of the actual settlement. That's not the case in England or Australia. We shouldn't ignore the lawyers' part in this disintegrating relationship between the profession and the public in America.

Brendan: No one is suggesting there should be a law telling doctors how to do an appendicectomy in 1978. For example, no one is saying where you should make your incision.

Chairman: Do you think the passage we have just considered would be a reasonable reply to the newspaper article?

Nicholas: No, I'm not sure I do. What the newspaper article said, or at least what Dr Burton said in his last paragraph, was that a doctor shouldn't have to be looking over his shoulder to see if what he's doing is the best for the patient and in accordance with the law. Now what the writer of this passage seems to be saying is that the doctors should be looking over their shoulders to the medical administrators and the specialists and the family doctor and so on.

Hilary: No; I don't see it that way. I see this passage making a plea for the doctor and all of these other people sitting around the table as equals. That's not to put the doctor in a God-like position but to have him consulting other people concerned with the case as an equal. It doesn't imply him looking over his shoulder at all. I don't think the doctor should be a puppet on a string as he would be if he was being dictated to by lawyers. In the *Medical Journal* passage, the doctor is making a common decision with other people.

Nicholas: Well, there are different sorts of laws and I suppose one could look at the *Medical Journal* passage and say it is recommending a sort of law when it says 'an ethical decision is not a task which is made easier by some external', etc. This passage itself tries to lay down an absolute. It doesn't say in some cases we'll do this and in others we'll do the opposite. It is saying what should be done in all cases.

Robert: You're twisting the point!

Chairman: Yes, I think the author of the passage is stating an opinion. It can't be seen in the same light as a law surely.

Nicholas: O.K. If the medical profession can function correctly without having what the rest of society has, that is, a legal stipulation as to its performance, if it can do that, that's absolutely perfect. But if it can't, then the purpose of laws is to ensure that we come as close as possible to that situation.

Chairman: Good. We are all agreed that we are disturbed by this sort of newspaper article appearing; that it is already a reflection on our professional performance; and that our goal should be to behave in a way which would negate the necessity for this sort of legislation.

[*General agreement.*]

Hilary: Absolutely.

David: I agree.

Gillian: Yes.

Rod: Yes.

Nicholas: Yes; but I wonder if this *is* the message we're taking away if we are leaving this table still thinking that we can make decisions about patients and yet not tell them the truth, or not tell them about aspects of their disease which affect them. I wonder if we really *are* taking that message away when some of us still believe we are entitled to that sort of breach of trust.

I started off today thinking that there would probably be many cases where I wouldn't tell the patient, but I am going to leave this session thinking that there are very few situations where that's the case.

Chairman: Have our attitudes changed or do they need to change? We are a traditionalist profession. There have been professional conventions that we don't always 'tell' the patients. Have times changed so that the patients are now better informed and want better information? Should our tendency be a little more towards the 'telling' school rather than the 'non-telling' school?

Gillian: I think there has been a change.

Colin: I think all patients want to be told if it's going to be beneficial to them provided it's not going to stuff things up as far as they're concerned.

Jane: I would just like to make a plea for the doctor working with the patient rather than as somebody above the patient. If that could be achieved a lot of this criticism of the profession wouldn't arise. Decisions to tell the patient something serious would then just be a natural flow-on from a healthy relationship which the doctor had with the patient.

Liz: Perhaps we should ask the patient do they want to know . . .

Rod [*laughing*]: Yeah, run up to the patient and say, 'Do you want to know if you've got cancer?'

Chairman: Rod, please let Liz finish!

Liz: Should we consider letting the patient make the decision about whether or not they want to be told . . .

Rod [*interrupting again*]: You can't. You can't go up to a patient and . . .

Chairman: Don't interrupt Rod, it's not fair! Let Liz finish.

Liz: Well I think you've got to feel your way around in your discussions with the patient, and then . . .

Rod [*interrupting again!*]: But you still have to make the decisions in the end yourself, after you've felt your way around with the patient.

Chairman: Rod, I can't hear what Liz is saying, and I'm not sure that anyone else can. Please let her finish!

Liz [*to Rod*]: Yes, shut up will you! [*Liz gives up trying to speak.*]

Nicholas: I completely agree with Liz. I think it is possible to spend some time with the patient before the point at which you are going to have to sit down and tell them something bad. I think perhaps we could ask the patient what they feel about this. I suppose it really is being hypothetical with the patient but you can ask, 'How would you react if the news was bad?'

Chairman: Both Liz and Nicholas have raised an interesting point. At the end of taking a history we don't routinely ask the patient, 'Well, if something bad was to crop up during this admission or during an investigation, would you or would you not want to know about it?' Should we?

David: I don't think it would be a matter of asking the patient, 'Do you want to be told?'; rather you would be asking them, 'How would you feel about that?' You can't ask a patient in the abstract because until he is confronted with it, I don't really think he'll know how he would respond.

Hilary: I would like to make a comment about having to say, 'How do you feel about it?' or 'Do you want to be told', to a patient who's in the ward before any investigations or diagnosis have been made. I think you should start with an open-ended discussion, as David suggests: talk about how they feel they would respond to such news, and in the end you will come to some conclusion as to how the best way would be to approach this patient.

Rod: If you do that, then you're disagreeing with Nick, because Nick was saying you shouldn't make any decisions on the patient without the patient's consent. But if you're talking about his feelings, then you've got to make the decision after you've assessed those feelings. The decision still finishes up with the doctor.

Chairman: What do you think the answer would be if you went down to the main street and asked a hundred people, 'If something serious cropped up in a hospital admission, would you want to be told?' What sort of answer do you think they'd give?

Gillian: I think most of them would say, 'Yes, I do want to know.'

Dave: I think you'd get a completely different set of replies from the people in the street than you would from those same people if they were in a hospital environment.

Chairman: So different as to make the question artificial and irrelevant?

Dave: Yes.

David: I think this business about asking the patient would they want to be told could be dangerous, because if the answer turns out to be 'No', you might have produced some sort of fear and doubt in their minds.

Stuart: This is one of the biggest problems facing a general practitioner. A patient may come in and the general practitioner may hunt around to find out if the patient does have cancer, especially if they have had some vague pains or something like that. Now that sort of patient may just want to be told that they don't have cancer, and the general practitioner is in the position of being almost certain that they don't, but can't definitely say it. There's always a doubt in his mind that there may be something further going on. Everytime a doctor says to a patient categorically, 'You're all right!', he runs the grave risk of being wrong.

Liz: The best way to overcome that is to make sure you're talking to the patient at each stage of the proceedings.

Chairman: On the other hand Liz, I wouldn't underestimate the size of the dilemma that Stuart has portrayed. It will be made easier by what you've said, but it won't be eliminated.

Nicholas: And yet you are not actually being a doctor if you're not asking yourself, '*Why* has this patient come to me with this particular problem?' Surely there must be something underlying the patient's pain.

Chairman: Nicholas, I think that's separate from the point which Stuart was making: given that many patients have a fear of cancer, the doctor may be in the difficult position of *wanting* to give a blanket reassurance to a patient with vague aches and pains, which the doctor feels (on the basis of the tests he's done and the examination he's made) are not due to anything serious—but still can't give a 100-per-cent assurance. The very qualification of that certainty, which all responsible doctors must make, may be enough to sow seeds of doubt and fear in a nervous patient's mind.

Stuart: Exactly.

Brendan: Going on from the point that Stuart just made, if the doctor did make a decision and advised the patient on the basis of his examination that he was all right, and then it turned out that he wasn't the doctor shouldn't feel bad. I don't think that is a reason the doctor should be looking over his shoulder.

Chairman: We seem to have gone through that thoroughly. To make sure we don't start going round in circles perhaps we might move on to a fresh topic: the use of patients in clinical experimental trials.

In this ethical week we could have discussed abortion, euthanasia, artificial insemination, genetic engineering, or some of the other common ethical issues, about which there has been a lot of debate and discussion. Instead I chose the issue of whether to 'tell' or 'not to tell' the patient. I really don't think it matters because the purpose of this week has been to highlight the structure and the apparatus with which we handle ethical problems, irrespective of which specific problem it is. In the eighteenth century, one of the major ethical issues was whether or not a doctor should attend the victims of duels—which were illegal. In the next century many of 'our' ethical issues will be just as dead.

I have tried not to impose my view of what your opinion should be on whether or not to tell the patient, instead I have seen it as my job to give you an idea of the complexity of all ethical issues.

Now, as our last topic for today, let's consider the issue of the use of patients in clinical trials. As a way in, could we quickly read four short passages.

Nathaniel Hawthorne, *The Scarlet Letter*

> In their researches into the human frame, it may be that the higher and more subtle faculties of [doctors] were materialised, and that they lost the spiritual view of existence amid the intricacies of that wondrous mechanism, which seemed to involve art enough to compass all of life within itself.[5]

Dr B. de Mandeville, *Fable of the Bees*

> Everybody knows, that surgeons in the cure of dangerous wounds and fractures, and the extirpation of Limbs, and other dreadful

> operations are often compelled to put their patients to extraordinary torments, and that the more desperate and calamitous cases occur to them, the more the outcries and bodily sufferings of others must become familiar for them; . . . their practice itself is sufficient to harden and extinguish in them that tenderness without which no man is capable of setting a true value upon the lives of his fellow creatures.[6]

H. G. Wells, *The Island of Dr Moreau*

> You cannot imagine what this means to an investigator, what an intellectual passion grows upon him. You cannot imagine the strange colourless delight of these intelligent desires. The thing before you is no longer an animal, a fellow creature, but a problem. . . . The study of Nature makes a man at last as remorseless as nature.[7]

G. B. Shaw, *Doctor's Dilemma*

> If the acquisition of knowledge justifies every sort of conduct, it justifies any sort of conduct . . . the exclusion of the pursuit of knowledge from the laws of honour is the most hideous conceivable enlargement of anarchy . . . the man who [does] it is ethically imbecile.[8]

Chairman: Does anyone want to comment on any of these passages?

Brendan: Yes, I would like to say a word about the Bernard Shaw passage. I think there's a truth in this passage. A lot of doctors see medicine as a branch of biology. They seem to be interested in the human body only as a collection of cells, and their whole attitude seems to be concerned with randomized controlled trials. They are obsessed with dividing patients into this group, that group, or the other. I think you have always got to keep in mind that the patient is a human being; and the laws of honour which he refers to are concerned more with the human being rather than the results of the experiments. The same thing applies to animal experimentation, you just can't chop animals about without giving consideration to what you're doing.

Hilary: I think there are a lot of doctors who are looking towards the results of clinical experimentation to improve cure rates and so on. Many of them are concerned with the quantity of life rather than the quality. This is especially so in something like breast cancer trials.

Stuart: I thought the passage from Hawthorne's novel expressed an interesting sentiment: that a lot of people in research become so preoccupied with what they're doing, and what they're getting into, that they almost lose their human existence and become materialized or materialists.

Rod: In a way that Hawthorne passage is right and wrong. I think for the average medical student, what we learn about the human body makes us feel more wondrous as to how it's all put together. But maybe in a way Stuart's right, that when you go too far, when you start delving into a minor detail like some research workers do, then you lose that view.

Gillian: I agree.

David: Yes, that's very true. When I first found out how D.N.A. worked [*laughter*], how all the intricacies of biochemistry worked, I sat back and thought, 'Well I don't really believe in God, but could all of this have happened accidentally?' It's just so amazing.

Dave: Just that it's all happened seems so incredible.

Gillian: On the other hand it often worries me that I am becoming hardened to people's suffering. For me it's the message in the second passage which is important–the one from Mandeville. We've been saying here today that people have to think of the patient's good and that you have to see the patient as a person, and that sort of thing. But I think it gets harder all the time, because you see so many patients and you see them suffering so much that you get to the point where it doesn't mean much any more. Maybe we are asking a lot of doctors to try and do both. Maybe that's why the profession is breaking down. The demands are too great.

Colin: I disagree, especially with the last sentence in the Mandeville passage. I don't believe that tenderness is necessarily extinguished or diminished. Cases do come to us which are 'desperate and calamitous', and if patients are going to continue to be sent to our hospitals or rooms we can't be the sort of person in whom tenderness is going to die out. I think patients would just stop coming.

Gillian: I think if you're too emotional or too involved, it is going to drain you.

Colin: No, it's not emotion.

David: This is what we discussed last week. It's the difference between purposeful emotion and useless pity.

Nicholas: I think we're over-generalizing. There are people who have become very hard and say, 'Oh, this suffering really doesn't mean anything', but it's not everybody by any means.

David: I agree, I think to an outsider a doctor's attempt to channel his emotions into something purposeful and something effective on the patient's behalf may look like callousness or indifference. I mean, when a doctor is concentrating on something he may seem indifferent.

Brendan: I don't think the practice of medicine exactly means you have to extinguish tenderness. What it does mean is that you have to pocket your mind to a certain extent. You can be tender and sympathetic when you are with a patient, and then forget about it as you move across to the next bed.

Chairman: Given that most of these passages are alluding to the use of patients in the context of furthering general scientific knowledge in clinical research, what are the dangers of this potential hardening (which Gillian says is inevitable) for the clinical research worker?

Brendan: He may lose the ability to look about a patient as a human being.

Stuart: That's right.

Brendan: A medical research worker cannot be a true scientist.. There are very few situations in medicine where you can have a pure scientific experiment

Chairman: What about the concept of consent?

Robert: I think that's sixteen years, isn't it?

Gillian [*not hearing Robert's joke*]*:* Quite often I reckon they don't know . . .

[*Raucous laughter.*]

Dave: Did you get that on the tape?

Gillian [*realizing what she said*]*:* Oh God, that's always happening!

Male student: Really Gillian?

Chairman [*after a pause*]*:* An inspired comment Robert! All right, now what about the problem of consent in relation to using patients in clinical research trials?

Gillian: I think most times it seems to be ignored.

Hilary: I think many patients think they're being treated when in fact they're being experimented on.

Chairman: Is it ever justified?

Rod: Yes, in double blind trials.

Chairman: Now wait a minute, what I am saying is that given you are going to do a double blind trial, would you ever neglect to sit down with the patient and explain to them that they were going to be put into a double blind trial, without necessarily telling them which side of the experiment they were going to be in.

Rod: Well, if you did that, that wouldn't really be a double blind trial, because the patient would be apprehensive about which group they were in.

Chairman: So you would waive the concept of consent in a double blind trial?

Rod: No, you're taking me too far, I didn't say that! What I am saying is that when you yourself do not know whether one thing is better than another . . .

Chairman: That is a different point.

David: If you are going to put the patient on any trial, you should explain if you are going to give them a new drug that it might work or it might not work. But you must tell them the truth.

Colin: I agree, I don't think Rod can get away with what he said . . .

Male student: He's got away with a hell of a lot today!

Colin [continuing]: You've either got to get consent, or they don't go into the trial. Now the doctor has got to make that decision. I would never put a patient on a clinical trial without their consent.

Chairman: Would anyone?

Rod: If you've got two drugs and you don't know the difference between them, you really don't know whether one is better than the other, so it doesn't really matter whether you tell the patient or not.

Nicholas [a groan].

Chairman: And what about the side-effects of these drugs or treatments? Are you going to subject the patient to them without their permission?

Stuart: Half the patients in this hospital seem to be on clinical trials without them knowing it.

Six students [trying to talk together].

Chairman: Stuart, you think that half the patients in this hospital who are on trials don't know it?

Rod: Every time you give a patient a dose of a drug, it's a sort of a trial.

Chairman: But the purely therapeutic situation is quite different from the use of a patient as a research subject. I think you have missed the point.

Dave: I don't think he has missed the point.

Colin: I do.

Chairman: I am saying that in any clinical trial, irrespective of the element of doubt, there is no excuse for not explaining to the trial subject the details of that trial. After all, it may not be of any direct therapeutic benefit to them at all. Let me make my position clear; what I am really asking you is this: would you ever use a human being as an experimental subject without him knowing about it?

Rod: Doesn't that happen all the time in medicine? Every time you say to the patient I am going to give you this drug, you don't know whether it's going to work or not.

Chairman: There is a great difference between using the consent for treatment which is implied in a patient knocking on your door and asking you to treat them, and extending that consent to the use of the same patient in a clinical trial which may be of no therapeutic benefit to them, and is really of interest to medical research and progress in general.

David: As long as this clinical trial you are putting them in isn't going to injure them in any way it wouldn't matter.

Chairman: Can you ever be sure, and who's going to make that decision?

David: Yes, well that's the big problem. On thinking about it it's hard to justify ever using a patient in a clinical trial without their permission.

Chairman: Can it be justified?

David: I can't think of any instance in which it would be justified. But I don't want to close my mind to the possibility that such a situation might occur.

Chairman: Well, could I say in conclusion on this point that there is no written medical code (as we know them) that will permit clinical experimentation without consent, and that no clinical trial has taken place in this hospital without the permission of the Ethics Committee. One of the clauses which has to be satisfied before that Committee will allow a trial to take place in this hospital is that the consent requirement must be fulfilled.

Dave: Does the patient actually have to sign a form?

Chairman: In many cases now that is true. It didn't used to be, written consent wasn't required, but in some institutes that is necessary now.

Liz: I think that's a good idea.

Stuart: I believe every resident doctor is a clinical trial.

[*Laughter.*]

Chairman: Stuart, I am grateful that you didn't say every consultant is. We are way past time already. This has been one of the most exciting sessions of the year. Thank you for your participation.

Liz: That really was an interesting topic. I enjoyed that!

Brendan: Yes, that really brought a lot of issues to light. A session like this can actually change your opinion. I'm convinced, I wasn't before, but I am much more convinced now that I am going to approach the patient much more openly in terms of what I tell them.

ESSAY 4

TRIALS OF TRUTH[1]

Of what use is genius, if the organ is too convex or too concave, and cannot find a focal distance within the actual horizon of human life?[2]
Ralph Waldo Emerson

In this chapter I would like to develop the theme on which we concluded the preceding session. It is so very important.

The discoveries of scientific medicine have contributed immeasurably to the excellence of our profession. At its best, science has a purity and excitement which few areas of human challenge can equal. At its most sublime, the discipline of science demands a quality of imaginative integration similar to that which is involved in the creation of a work of art. Science expresses so much of the richest potential of the human mind in which personal satisfaction can be harmonized with social good. The best science is hard work for it involves great patience, attention to detail, ingenuity, and, above all, imagination.

Yet there are dangers against which scientific workers in clinical practice must stand on guard. Any medical research which involves human beings places the scientific worker in a position of potential compromise and can confront him with moral dilemmas. The thoughts which follow do not in any way express a cynical view of science–quite the opposite. I would like to feel that they would be endorsed by all scientists who are concerned with both the scientific significance and the total integrity of their work. There are dangers associated with clinical experimentation.

All doctors and nurses know that there are occasions when nothing but despair and degradation comes from telling the complete truth to a patient. However true this is in *clinical* practice I feel very strongly that this in no way justifies any liberty taken with the concept of truth when explaining details to a patient who is being asked to take part in a *research* trial. This is especially so when the benefit to the patient is doubtful or indirect. Here the guidelines are clear. In both the 1964 Helsinki resolution on clinical trials, and the National Health and Medical Research Council's statement of 1973, the absolute requirement of the patient's concent is underlined. It is not enough for the doctor to make a mental calculation and decide that, on balance, the patient will receive more benefit than risk. The consent for treatment which is implied by a patient asking a doctor to care for him should not be taken as consent for participation in a clinical trial.

There is a paradox at the heart of the ethical exercise which deals with clinical research studies. We have two major interests to serve in performing research: the potential benefits to the public, and the rights of the individual patient or volunteer. To some extent these interests are in competition. It must be an absolute rule that if there is any indication of unwillingness to participate, the patient should not be included in the trial. The patient's *informed* consent is necessary in *all* cases. Assumed consent, consent under any persuasion whatsoever, or consent achieved from those in dependent or vulnerable positions, is absolutely void.

While it is probably true that the over-zealous interpretation of the concept of consent could cause virtually all clinical trials to grind to a halt, this should not deter us from extreme vigilance in our own attitude towards consent.

If consent cannot be obtained because the explanation of what is going to be done is either too scientific, too inhumane, too delicate, or too difficult (as in the case of foreign, confused, or simple patients), then the research trial should exclude that person. In other words, if for any reason informed consent cannot be obtained our tendency should be not to go ahead, rather than to bend our concept of consent, or to encourage laxity in our ideal of consent. We cannot afford to shrug our moral shoulders over clinical experimentation. Although some will disagree, I believe that what is morally wrong cannot be scientifically valid. Nor is a dubious clinical trial made ethical by a result which is scientifically interesting or clinically rewarding.

Acknowledging that there is a potential conflict between the rights of the society and medical research on one hand, and the rights of our patients on the other, our conviction should always be that the rights of patients must take priority. Coercion, or the exploitation of our position of trust, are absolutely alien to the conduct of clinical trials. It hardly needs to be said that once consent has been achieved there should be no decrease in the vigilance with which the trial is conducted, and no reduction in the research worker's responsibility for all that happens.

The problem of consent really is one of judgement and delicacy, for irrespective of the guidelines put forward by an ethics committee, the success of any system will depend ultimately on the integrity of the individual doctors concerned. There can be no perfect system when humans are dealing with human issues. As members of the human family, doctors share the blemishes of the breed. Even so, the sentiment expressed by the International Code of Medical Ethics which was adopted by the World Medical Association, gives us encouragement: 'As a Stream cannot rise above its source, so a code cannot change a low-grade man into a high-grade doctor, but it can help a good man to be a better man and a more enlightened doctor. It can quicken and inform a conscience, but not create one.'[3]

Nowhere is the moral maxim that 'the good things a man can do are made complete only by the things he refuses to do' better applied than in relation to clinical trials. The most difficult task a doctor faces in relation to his prospective trial patient is to make the imaginative leap needed to realize what it is to be the specific patient who is sitting beside him. He must imagine the patient asking, 'Just who is it that you are doing this for?' and must be able to answer openly.

Socrates believed that knowledge, wisdom, happiness, and moral virtue were related absolutely. A good man was a wise man, and a wise man was always a happy man. Such a sublimity is beyond most of us. As clinical research workers, we face many ethical situations where we are forced to choose between knowledge and morality—in opposition to the long-standing sentiment that the two must go together.

The idea of consent does not imply the open-endedness of ethical discussions in general. Let us consider the relationship between the concepts of consent and of ethical problems.

During the last session a passage of my own was discussed which made the following points: clinical trials and clinical practice can both involve difficult ethical problems—tasks which are not made easier by some legislative dictate telling doctors what they *ought* to do. Such rules are alien to the nature of medical practice and ethical decisions, both of which are influenced by the circumstances and opinions of individual patients and doctors. Such decisions should be joint verdicts involving the patient, the family doctor, the specialist, medical administrators, and—when the adult patient so desires—his family. They should consider not only purely medical evidence, but the resources of the family and the patient (economic, emotional, psychological, and physical), as well as the ethical issues involved. In contrast to these ethical issues, it is the patient alone who decides if he is willing to give consent to be used in a research trial.

Those concerned with ethical issues are aware of three facets in the nature of the ethical process. First, that unlike strictly scientific questions, there is no current consensus of what is held to be a truth, and proof is not the ultimate warrant of truth. In the last analysis the answers to ethical questions are problematical. Second, that ethical problems cannot be considered in a void divorced from the whole historical and philosophical tradition of moral philosophy. And third, that ethical problems require a different form of thought to that which is applied to scientific problems (which may themselves be involved as one factor in the ethical equation); for they must consider the patient's rights, and in particular his right to be illogical, capricious, whimsical, sentimental, or even prejudiced. Only the third is closely related to the concept of consent.

In society as we know it, and according to medical codes and guidelines, to deny the patient his right to refuse consent is wrong. According to our present beliefs, society, science, or the self-fulfilment of the research worker, are irrelevant to the issue of consent.

On any specific ethical issue a number of different truths may be held by a doctor or the patient. They could, for example, subscribe to an absolute and inflexible moral belief such as the sanctity of life and denial of any means which would end a life. For them life is the absolute warrant of ethical judgement. An antagonist could rebuke this opinion but he could not refute it. He could order his own moral decisions according to other beliefs, but he could not undermine the validity of such an opinion held in full conscience. On the other hand other persons could regard the quality of living as their guiding belief, and might hold a much more flexible attitude towards the sanctity of life. The prolongation of life at any cost would seem to them—and they could be doctors, nurses, patients, or relatives—to be an ethical error.

Now while it is in the nature of ethical discussions that with two such divergent principles there must be mutual respect for their two offspring opinions, and not just a perfunctory lipservice for the right of others to hold a polar view, and while ethics asks for a real conviction that opponents have an equal chance of holding an ethically valid opinion, the idea of consent implies that it is the patient alone who decides. In our society the concept of consent is outside ethics, for adult patients do not have to agree, and children should not be made to agree to be research subjects.

Another danger which can creep into clinical experimentation is to justify any practice by claiming that we are doing it for what we are convinced is a *good* motive, or a *good* end. But such reasoning can justify *any* action. As I mentioned in the last session we need to keep in mind that moral actions can be considered from four points of view; the motivation, the principle, the method or means, and the consequence. To rely exclusively on any single moral parameter can produce all sorts of horrible moral results. In the last session I offered some examples: if a person subscribed absolutely to the morality of *motivation*, then *any* act could be justified on the basis of 'well, I thought it was for good'. Exclusive adherence to the code of moral *consequence*, as we saw, would fail to differentiate between the unwitting and the deliberate transmission of plague to a population. Clearly, such fractionation of the individual elements of the moral milieu is theoretically artificial and practically ludicrous. In any moral situation all these elements, and many others—such as the specific needs appropriate to the patient or situation, the written and unwritten moral ordinances which operate in society, and current public feeling–must be considered and counterpoised. This is what makes the moral weave so challenging, so difficult, and occasionally so desperate.

Frequently in a clinical trial it is the most junior member involved–a medical student or a nurse–who has the purest and simplest view of the total moral mixture. It is he who feels the disquiet about what is being done which most accurately captures the concern of the patients, or the would-be concern of the patients had all of the facts been explained while their consent was being sought.

There will come a time in dealing with patients when doctors and nurses 'must in a greater measure become moral philosophers, asking themselves some quite profound questions about the nature of proper moral reasoning, and how moral dilemmas are rightly to be resolved'.[4]

As human beings we have an almost infinite talent to mislead ourselves and others about the nature of our activities. Indeed, they are so frequent, these evasions and moral side-steps, that one wonders whether they are essential for our human well-being. Perhaps the fundamental human paradox in which *our moral capacity always falls short of our moral ideal*, needs the buffer of our moral shuffles to enable us to live with our common shortcomings.

But nowhere is this more dangerous and inappropriate than in relation to our responsibilities to patients of whom we are asking special consent.

SESSION 5

HINDRANCES TO COMMUNICATION

Chairman: In the first session of our course we considered the patient's experience of illness, and in the second our discussion was concerned with the relatives. In Session 3 we noted the way doctors have been portrayed in literature, and last week we considered the framework of ethical discussions. This week we shall try and bring these first four sessions together in a consideration of clinical communication.

All medical activities–research, administration, academic and clinical–have as their common end point a patient who is trying to communicate a symptom or an anxiety to a doctor who is trying to alleviate them.

Could we start by considering a passage from Virginia Woolf's novel, *Mrs Dalloway*.

> Nothing could arouse him. Rezia put him to bed. She sent for . . . Dr Holmes. Dr Holmes examined him. There was nothing whatever the matter, said Dr Holmes. Oh, what a relief! What a kind man, what a good man! thought Rezia. When he felt like that he went to the Music Hall, said Dr Holmes. He took a day off with his wife and played golf. Why not try two tabloids of bromide dissolved in a glass of water at bedtime? These old Bloomsbury houses, said Dr Holmes, tapping the wall, are often full of very fine panelling, which the landlords have the folly to paper over. Only the other day, visiting a patient. Sir Somebody Something, in Bedford Square–.
>
> . . .
>
> Dr Holmes came again. Large, flesh-coloured, handsome, flicking his boots, looking in the glass, he brushed it all aside–headaches, sleeplessness, fears, dreams–nerve symptoms and nothing more, he said. If Dr Holmes found himself even half a pound below eleven stone six, he asked his wife for another plate of porridge at breakfast. (Rezia would learn to cook porridge.) But, he continued, health is largely a matter in our own control. Throw

yourself into outside interests; take up some hobby. He opened Shakespeare–*Anthony and Cleopatra*; pushed Shakespeare aside. Some hobby, said Dr Holmes, for did he not owe his own excellent health (and he worked as hard as any man in London) to the fact that he could always switch off from his patients on to old furniture? And what a very pretty comb, if he might say so, Mrs Warren Smith was wearing!

When the damned fool came again, Septimus refused to see him . . .[1]

Chairman: Who would like to open the discussion?

Tony: I can understand Holmes's approach, but I think it's inadequate. He has a very narrow idea of what is medically significant. He considers there's nothing wrong with a patient if there's no physical illness. He seems to have the attitude of a human being who is healthy looking down on someone whom he considers 'functional', saying, 'Go on, get out, get a few interests!' and so on. After he has decided there's nothing organically wrong with the patient he adopts a non-medical role. He dismisses the patient's concerns.

David: I think this Holmes sounds a little like Dr Tyrell in the passage from Somerset Maugham's novel . . .

Chairman: You were fairly favourably disposed towards Dr Tyrell if I remember David?

David: No, I've changed my mind about him since then. [*Laughter.*] I think Holmes is a bit of a twit! He seems to say [*speaking with exaggerated emphasis*], 'Because *I'm* all right, because *I* don't have any nerve symptoms, it's silly for anyone else to have them, how can anyone else *possibly* have problems.' It's a superb last line–'When the damned fool came again, Septimus refused to see him'. I'm very sympathetic to that. The doctor has obviously done nothing for him. He has just used the visit as some sort of ego trip.

Rod: I'm not sure when this passage was written . . .

Chairman: About 1920 . . .

Rod: Yes. Well about the time it was written, this was the approach which was expected from doctors. It's only recently that we have begun to think about the human side of medical problems.

Tony: I think the opposite is the case. Medical men in the past were considered to have a much more wide-ranging role both in the community and in their medical approach. It's only in the last twenty or thirty years that scientism has been so exclusively applied to medicine.

Colin: I agree with Tony.

Chairman: You've seized on the purely medical aspect of the case. Is there any other?

Hilary: This doctor brushes over the medical aspects of the case just as fast as he can, and then he seems more at ease talking about golf or the music hall or anything else he can think of. Another point is that he talks to the wife and relates to her (at least *she* thinks he does); the patient is ignored and doesn't seem to have achieved any benefit from what is going on.

Colin: I agree, he hasn't addressed himself to the patient at all. He seems just to be talking to the wife.

David: There's not much of a medical case here anyway, it's more like a psychiatric case.

Chairman: It does say he has headaches, sleeplessness, and fears–on these symptoms this man could have an early brain tumour.

David: I agree. But Holmes's interpretation is that it's not a strictly medical case.

Chairman: How would you score Dr Holmes as a communicator?

Brendan: I think he has the sort of manner which wouldn't allow the patient to say anything. He seems to talk on in his own pontificating manner, and then is out through the door before the patient has had a chance to say anything to him. I don't think he would be much good at all; although, as we said before, there may be the odd patient who would like this sort of approach. He's come into the house and said quite a lot: he says, 'I'm all right', and 'When I feel like that I go to the music hall', and 'Throw yourself into other interests'–his approach is very superficial. He doesn't concern himself with the patient at all. He hasn't seen the problem from the patient's point of view.

Robert: He seems to say, 'I haven't got these complaints, and neither should you'. Or, 'If I get them, I can get rid of them, and so should you.'

David: He's almost using the patient's own plight to reinforce his own feelings that *he's* all right.

Gillian: I don't think you can communicate with somebody unless you've got some understanding of their needs. He doesn't seem to be even trying.

Rod: The part that caught me was when his wife says, 'What a relief! what a kind man, what a good man'. It seems that as soon as the doctor says that there is nothing wrong with the patient the wife thinks of the doctor as God.

Hilary: I think the wife *has* put the doctor on a pedestal, and it's reinforcing the sort of behaviour which Brendan was pointing out and which we don't like. The fact that she's looking at him in awe makes him feel he can go on getting away with what he's doing.

Nicholas: I don't think he takes himself down to the level of the patient . . .

Robert [*with a grin*]: You mean *up* to the patient?
Nicholas [*smiling*]: Yes. He's obviously very frightened.
Chairman: Do you think Dr Holmes has sufficient insight to know that his performance is shoddy? What do you think his response would be to the fact that Septimus refused to see him the next time?
Robert: He would just call the patient a silly so-and-so, and would probably criticize the patient.
David: I don't think he would be terribly upset at all.
Chairman: There's a lilting insolence about this fellow, isn't there? He comes into the patient's home, gives the floorboards and the skirting a bit of a tap, preens himself in front of the mirror, and then has the audacity to comment on the 'very pretty comb' that the patient's wife is wearing. On top of all that he advises the patient to get a hobby, at the very same moment that he pushes his patient's hobby–Shakespeare–aside.
Hilary: He's probably just looking forward to getting back to Sir Somebody Something or other–whose name he can't remember either.
Chairman: So no one has anything good to say about Holmes?
David: I'm sure he'd be a good bloke down at the club.

[*Laughter.*]

Chairman: Well now, let's go on and consider the next passage; it's from the same book. Septimus gets referred to Sir William Bradshaw who is a neurology specialist. This is the longest passage we consider in the course, but as much of it is dialogue I don't think it's too difficult to read.

> Sir William himself was no longer young. He had worked very hard; he had won his position by sheer ability (being the son of a shop-keeper), loved his profession; made a fine figurehead at ceremonies and spoke well–all of which had by the time he was knighted given him a heavy look, a weary look (the stream of patients being so incessant, the responsibilities and privileges of his profession so onerous), which weariness, together with his grey hairs, increased the extraordinary distinction of his presence and gave him the reputation (of the utmost importance in dealing with nerve cases) not merely of lightning skill and almost infallible accuracy in diagnosis, but of sympathy; tact; understanding of the human soul.
>
> He could see the first moment they came into the room. . . . It was a case of complete breakdown–complete physical and nervous breakdown, with every symptom in an advanced stage, he ascertained in two or three minutes (writing answers to questions, murmured discreetly, on a pink card) . . .

It was merely a question of rest, said Sir William; of rest, rest, rest; a long rest in bed. There was a delightful home down in the country where her husband would be perfectly looked after. . . .

'We have had our little talk,' said Sir William.

'He says you're very, very ill,' Rezia cried.

'We have been arranging that you should go into a home,' said Sir William.

'One of Holmes's homes?' sneered Septimus.

The fellow made a distasteful impression. For there was in Sir William . . . who had never had time for reading, a grudge, deeply buried, against cultivated people who came into his room and intimated that doctors, whose profession is a constant strain upon all the highest faculties, are not educated men . . .

'We all have our moments of depression,' said Sir William.

Once you fall, Septimus repeated to himself, human nature is on you. Holmes and Bradshaw are on you. They scour the desert. They fly screaming into the wilderness. The rack and the thumbscrew are applied. Human nature is remorseless.

'Impulses came upon him sometimes?' Sir William asked, with his pencil on a pink card.

That was his own affair, said Septimus.

'Nobody lives for himself alone,' said Sir William, glancing at the photograph of his wife in Court dress. 'And you have a brilliant career before you,' said Sir William. There was Mr Brewer's letter on the table. 'An exceptionally briliant career.' . . .

'I–I–' he stammered.

'Yes?' Sir William encouraged him. (But it was growing late.)

'I–I–' Septimus stammered.

'Try to think as little about yourself as possible,' said Sir William kindly. Really, he was not fit to be about.

Was there anything else they wished to ask him? Sir William would make all arrangements (he murmured to Rezia) and he would let her know between five and six that evening.

'Trust everything to me,' he said, and dismissed them. Never, never had Rezia felt such agony in her life! She had asked for help and been deserted! He had failed them! Sir William Bradshaw was not a nice man. . . . But what more did she want? . . .

To his patients he gave three-quarters of an hour; and if in this exacting science which has to do with what, after all, we know nothing about–the nervous system, the human brain–a doctor loses his sense of proportion, as a doctor he fails. Health we must have; and health is proportion. . . .

Proportion, divine proportion, Sir William's goddess, was acquired by Sir William walking hospitals, catching salmon, begetting one son in Harley Street by Lady Bradshaw, who caught salmon herself and took photographs scarcely to be distinguished from the work of professionals. Worshipping proportion, Sir William not only prospered himself but made England prosper, secluded her lunatics, forbade childbirth, penalised despair, made it impossible for the unfit to propagate their views until they, too, shared his sense of proportion—his, if they were men, Lady Bradshaw's if they were women.[2]

Rod: Bradshaw's attitude seems to change through the passage. At the start the author seems to indicate that Sir William is kind and generous, and is very talented. The opening suggests that he's warm to these people. And yet, at the end, in the last sentence, he seems to say that no one is really normal until they agree with his views.

Colin: I don't think it changes.

Gillian: No, neither do I.

Colin: I think he imagines himself to be a sympathetic, hardworking doctor, but at the same time he's 'hung-up' about himself being a person on whom others should model themselves. The same could be said about the way he sees his wife.

Rod: I wasn't saying that the doctor actually changes, I was saying that the author's opinion of him changes.

David: I don't agree that the author's attitude changes either. I think the first paragraph is being cynical, it's obviously tongue in cheek. I think Bradshaw is being set up completely for what is going to come. The author doesn't really want us to believe he's a fine figurehead or that he embodies extraordinary distinction.

Hilary: There is a very distinct difference between the first paragraph, where we are given a portrait of the impression the doctor would like to think he makes in public, and the following paragraphs where there is a movement to the actual view that the patient has of his performance.

David: I think this is a good portrait of a doctor's self-deception. He would really like to feel that 'the stream of patients is incessant and that the responsibilities and privileges of his profession so onerous', but the author certainly is not taken in.

Jane: It also says that he ascertained the symptoms in two or three minutes.

Rod: But later we are told he takes forty-five minutes with his patients. I think that's a very reasonable time for a doctor to take with a patient. Most of us would feel that we would have some idea of what is going on in the first two or three minutes; after all, the first question we ask is, 'What did you come into hospital for?'

Chairman: On the other hand, the point Jane mentioned might be the first indication in the passage that we should hold some reservation about this doctor's performance. What do you feel about that last paragraph? Is its tone and technique unexpected and abrupt in the context of the whole passage?

Nicholas: Early in the passage the author is more or less hinting at these defects in Bradshaw. But at the end, it becomes absolutely candid and direct.

Rod: With statements like 'secluded her lunatics', 'penalised despair', and 'made it impossible for the unfit to propagate their views', and so on, she really is quite hostile towards this doctor. I must admit that I didn't read it at first with as much insight as David in relation to the irony of the first paragraph. But when I reached the last paragraph I realized that he was probably sending his patient off to an asylum. It wasn't just a little rest home.

Tony: I think in the last paragraph Virginia Woolf is intruding into the passage. She seems to be intruding all of her own hang-ups and all of her discontentment with the sort of medical treatment she feared.

Chairman: I agree Tony. Some people, for example Henry James, would say that this last paragraph is bad writing in that the author has walked on to her page and is making direct pronouncements. In other words she's *telling* us about Bradshaw rather than *showing* us what he is like—as she did in the early part of the passage. One of the students in an earlier group said that he felt the last paragraph jolted and was neither as subtle nor as good as the technique of writing in the early part of the passage. When an author intrudes it disrupts the reader's feeling that the book is a harmonious work of fiction. Suddenly we are confronted with a lecture which destroys the aesthetic blend.

Gillian: I see what you mean.

Could I come back to Bradshaw. I don't think it's that easy because I believe we could all be guilty of the same sort of medical behaviour. I mean, if we're preoccupied with what's going on in the patient we may appear to be distant. I'm not saying that excuses it, but it might make us look on it a little more charitably.

Brendan: There seem to be a lot of Bradshaws walking around in the medical profession, in the sense of someone who really thinks that his performance is good when in fact it's bad . . .

Chairman: Well, as Rod said, Sir William Bradshaw did spend forty-five minutes with the patient; he did take the initiative in arranging the new hospital; and he did say, 'Leave everything to me'—in other words he *did* accept responsibility for the management of the patient . . .

Brendan [*continuing*]: That was the point I was coming to. I think there are a lot of patients who are satisfied with the Bradshaws of the world. And for those patients his lack of insight isn't readily apparent; they've got their own preoccupations and miss the sensitive issues which are portrayed here. As Tony said of Virginia Woolf, she obviously had seen Bradshaws and had been frustrated by his sort of attitude.

Nicholas: I don't think it's just a specific attack on the Bradshaws, it's a more general attack on the society which surrounds him. She is attacking a system of values, and Bradshaw is really the ultimate or perfect product of that system of values. He's a self-made man, he's working for society, and he's doing what society would want. He seems to be trying to make 'little Bradshaws' out of all his patients. It's very much an 'anti-individuality' sort of approach. He's just making people into what he feels society would want them to be.

Tony: These sort of defects can arise in anybody who sees their job as propping up the sanity of society. I believe the questions are so complex and so involved that it would be only an incredible person who could make the decisions involved, without undergoing a lot of self-doubt and self-criticism. It would seem that Sir William doesn't possess the self-judgement necessary for a man who is trying to do what he is doing.

Chairman: What do you think could have been the possible evolution of this man? How can we explain some of the blemishes you have identified in his performance?

Colin: I think he's come up the hard way and he's had to fight for what he's got.

Gillian: Perhaps he knew someone else like that, who was his ideal, and on whom he modelled himself–I mean someone who was prominent in the profession. Bradshaw has become attracted to the more social aspects of being a doctor and I think that could have contributed to his performance. On the other hand I think he's a little bit jealous of the more cultured or sophisticated aspects of society–I think he says somewhere that he had a grudge, deeply buried, against cultivated people. He felt deficient in that area. He's probably more interested in bettering himself than he is in giving medical service.

Chairman: Does the communication between the doctor and the patient deteriorate as the passage goes on?

Brendan: I don't think it was ever there.

Colin: I think it was there, actually. He has obviously talked to the patient and talked to his wife. But once he has told Septimus what he plans to do, he seems to be saying, 'Well, I've talked to this patient, but it's all the same anyway, there's not much to do, it's merely a question of rest.'

Rod: I don't see anywhere where he had a really good conversation with the patient.

Colin: Well, I assumed he did from the fact that he's been with him for forty-five minutes.

Jane: I think the communication with the wife deteriorates, but I don't think there was really ever any good communication between Sir William and Septimus.

Rod: It's interesting that, in the previous passage, the wife heard what she wanted to hear and thought Holmes was a good doctor and a nice man and so on; but at the end of this passage she is saying that she had never felt such agony in her life, she'd been deserted, he had failed them, and that Sir William was not a nice man. She becomes less gullible.

Chairman: Where in the passage is there an indication that Sir William did desert the patient?

Brendan: It comes at the end of Septimus's comment, ' "One of Holmes's homes?" ' The passage then continues–'The fellow made a distasteful impression.' From then on things get bad because the patient is rejecting this therapy.

Nicholas: No; I think you could point to it even earlier than that: where Sir William says, 'It's merely a question of rest, rest, rest.' That really seems to devalue the patient's whole illness.

Tony: I believe that there could have been deception on the part of Sir William. I mean, if he *is* putting Septimus into an asylum, there's a good deal more involved than rest. There could be restraint, and drugs, and so on.

Hilary: Even taking it literally as rest, it's still condescending and dismissive.

Tony: But even before that, it says that Sir William has had a little talk with Septimus's wife. They have bypassed the patient. He's told the patient's wife that he's very, very ill but he hasn't sat down and talked to Septimus about it. I think there has been a patronizing attitude towards Septimus right from the outset.

Hilary: And Septimus says, 'And once you fall human nature is upon you'. He seems to be both vulnerable and excluded. He has no say in it.

Chairman: Why do you think Sir William's performance was less than perfect?

Jane: Well I think in the first paragraph we get a clue where it says 'the stream of patients being so incessant, the responsibilities and privileges of his profession so onerous'. Also, he is a senior man and he has had to work very hard to get where he is: he is a success. That may not make him very tolerant of people who are different to himself and who haven't succeeded against the odds, or who can't climb up the ladder.

Chairman: I like Jane's point: the fact that Sir William has never failed (he's always been on top of it with his knighthood and his position at the pinnacle of the profession), might make him less tolerant towards poor Septimus, who certainly has fallen and who feels that the world is now upon him.

Rod: I think the society he has been brought up in and the medical system he has been working in wouldn't help him understand somebody like Septimus.

Colin: He's got preconceived ideas of how people should behave. They should behave like him.

Tony: Yes, the authority of the medical profession is always suspect when they are not dealing with physical illness. They're at their most powerful when there are not too many questions to be asked. But with areas which are still in considerable doubt, where there are a lot of questions to be asked, there, an authoritarian attitude like Sir William's is very open to question.

Chairman: Was there any moment in this passage where Septimus looked like he was going to speak up? And what was the response from Sir William?

Gillian: I think at the point where Septimus stammers ' "I–I–" ' and after that Sir William says ' "Try to think as little about yourself as possible" '.

Chairman: Some of you may remember in Session 1 when Hilary said that a lot of patients feel that their worries are passed over and missed by a doctor who is preoccupied with the specific medical aspects of the case. I think the patient often comes with a worry that frequently isn't articulated early on in the interview and is only mentioned as a parting comment. If a doctor misses the patient's particular concern, the patient becomes far less interested in all that the doctor has to say to him from then on. Not infrequently, when, at a later date, a patient says to the doctor, 'You didn't tell me that', and the doctor *has* told the patient, it's because the doctor himself was inattentive to what the patient was trying to say. The patient's response to that indifference is simply to tune out from the whole medical interview, and in taking no further interest they don't hear what the doctor is saying to them.

All right. Are you feeling a little bit flat after last week's hectic discussion?

Gillian: No, it's just so damn' hot today!

Chairman: Well let's have a look at a short poem now, for a change. It's called 'For A Journey'—and it's by Alan Brownjohn who is a contemporary English poet. Read it to the rhythm of its punctuation.

House Field, Top Field, Oak Field, Third Field:
Though maps conclude their duties, the names trek on
Unseen across every county. Farmers call hillocks
And ponds and streams and lanes and rocks
By the first words to hand; a heavy, whittled-down
Simplicity meets the need, enough to help say
Where has yielded best, or the way they walked from home.
You can travel safely over land so named—
Where there is nowhere that could not somewhere
Be found in a memory which knows, and loves.

So watch then, all the more carefully, for
The point where the pattern ends: where mountains, even,
And swamps and forests and gaping bays acquire
The air of not needing ever to be spoken of.

Who knows what could become of you where
No one has understood the place with names?[3]

Chairman: Who likes this poem?

Brendan: It's a poem that expresses an affection for the simplicity of things, particularly names. It's hard to put my feeling about this poem into words, but it's basically asking us to be aware of the meaning behind certain names—especially names which have an intrinsic quality, those which require understanding.

Nicholas: I like it because it seems to set down a true separation between the known and the unknown aspect of things. I got the impression that he may have been talking about the journey of death in the last part—the final journey.

Jane: I liked it too. To some extent I saw it as a warning against taking things too superficially—not to take things on their face value.

David: This poem certainly is more than it appears on the surface. It is much more than a poem about what fields are called.

Chairman: Do you think there's a philosophy in the poem?

David: Yes, I think it's trying to indicate the apparent safety of familiarity, and the threat of the unknown.

Gillian: I agree, I like it very much.

Tony: I like it too. Perhaps it's a poem about labels and about categories in general. Underlying it is a criticism of systems which simplify things by categorization. It is just as David said, there's safety in familiarity.

Brendan: That's why some people have an affection for rigidity. There's a message here for a lot of doctors.

Chairman: I get that sense from the poem too, especially in the lines 'So watch then, all the more carefully, for / The point where the pattern ends'. Does the poem create a mood that makes you feel threatened when you move into this area?

Hilary: I think it's a warning more than a threat.

Brendan: I don't see it so much as a warning, I think there's almost an invitation involved in this poem. It's an area that everyone should wander into at some time.

Chairman: I feel the same. It seems to be part of the challenge of being a human being to accept the excitement of uncertainty.

Now let's move from this poem which directed us towards 'words' to a passage from Lewis Carroll's *Through the Looking Glass.*

'I don't know what you mean by "glory" ', Alice said.

Humpty Dumpty smiled contemptuously. 'Of course you don't—till I tell you. I meant "there's a nice knock-down argument for you!" '

'But "glory" doesn't mean a nice knock-down argument'—Alice objected.

'When *I* use a word,' Humpty Dumpty said in rather a scornful tone, 'it means just what I choose it to mean—neither more nor less.'

'The question is,' said Alice, 'whether you can make words mean different things.'

'The question is,' said Humpty Dumpty, 'which is to be master—that's all.'[4]

Chairman: I suppose that's why they couldn't put Humpty back together again—no one could understand his symptoms. Does this passage have any medical relevance?

Students: Yes.

Rod: Last week someone quoted the example of a woman who was told she had a tumour and she responded with, 'Oh well, I'm glad I haven't got cancer.' A doctor can use words but the patient doesn't understand them unless both people attach the same meaning to the word.

Robert: It's a similar thing when we ask the patient do they have a cough, and they say no. Then they cough and you say, 'What's that?' and they say, 'It's just clearing my throat.' Some patients feel they have only got to cough if they are coughing something up.

Chairman: What about the problem of using technical words in medical communication?

Liz: In some ways it's advantageous, in other ways it's not. It can be advantageous if it allows a doctor to talk in front of the patient without alarming them unduly by using words which they don't understand, or which, at that moment, aren't relevant to their particular problem. On the other hand, technical medical words may be confused or misinterpreted by the patient when a doctor is speaking directly to them.

Jane: Another drawback of using technical medical terms is that it makes the patient feel they are below the doctor, and so it hinders good communication. If the doctor knows what these technical words mean and the patient doesn't, there is immediate alienation. The patient has no way of dealing with that. It could make the patient scared of the doctor. To sensitive patients it could indicate that the doctor just doesn't want to talk to them. In using a bad choice of words he could stimulate a communication breakdown.

Hilary: Even when a doctor is aware of Jane's point, and *is* trying not to use technical words, he often doesn't realize which level to aim at for the patient who is in front of him. He might think he's doing the right thing and still not be understood.

David: I often feel inadequate when I'm trying to explain something to my non-medical friends. They reply with, 'Well what does that mean?' When you try to explain a medical concept, you realize just how condescending you sound.

Gillian: And when we talk to people who don't understand English well, we often raise our voice, as though shouting at them is going to improve their understanding. Sometimes you are not even aware you're doing it.

Rod: I think another important area is the difficulty of communicating between doctors, especially medical students trying to communicate with doctors. I know in my last medical term I asked three different consultants what they meant by 'stony dullness', and they all told me something different.

Liz: Frequently in medicine everyone has their own concept of what a word means and sometimes there are different understandings of the same medical concept.

Chairman: We've discussed the advantages and disadvantages of using technical medical terms, and Liz just mentioned the idea of words with common meanings having different meanings to different people. What are some of these?

Tony: Indigestion.

Robert: Pain.

Tony: Giddiness.

Chairman: Good. Now most of those have a medical connotation, but what about everyday words that are used and which have specific medical meaning?

Gillian: Complications.

Male student: Palpitations.

Chairman: What about 'acute' and 'chronic'? [*Agreement.*] Or the words 'theatre' or 'follow-up' or 'work-up' or 'special test' or 'history'?

Liz: Oh, I see what you mean: words which doctors use in a specific way but which normal people use with the ordinary meaning.

Chairman: Yes; let me give an example. I was once on a ward round where an elderly lady, who had an inoperable cancer of the breast, was being discussed. When a surgeon was asked what he planned, he said he was going to do a 'toilet operation'. Now *we* all know that means just an operation for hygiene; but I was looking at the patient's face when this was said and I am sure, elderly lady that she was, she thought that she was going to be taken off down to the lavatory to be operated on! [*Laughter.*] Then again we have normal words which have different meanings to different people. They can be a problem in a medical communication too. Let me illustrate what I mean by the passage from Virginia's Woolf's essay 'On Being Ill'.

> English, which can express the thoughts of Hamlet, or the tragedy of Lear, has no words for the shiver and the headache. It has all grown one way. The merest schoolgirl, when she falls in love, has Shakespeare or Keats to speak her mind for her; but let the sufferer try to describe a pain in his head to a doctor and the language runs dry. There is nothing ready for him. He is forced to coin words himself, and, taking his pain in one hand, and a lump of pure sound in the other . . . crush them together that a brand new word in the end drops out.[5]

Liz: Yes, 'pain' can be a problem. But I think it's up to the doctor to ask the patient just exactly what they mean, and, if they're having difficulty, for the doctor to give the patient some words with which they can express themselves. [*General disagreement.*] Hmmm, I suppose that could lead to even greater confusion. It could interfere with the patient's interpretation of their pain.

Nicholas: This brings up another point: even when we take away all the technical terms, and even with the best intent, it's still very, very hard to communicate something which is within you and which doesn't really lend itself to words.

Liz: You certainly could say the same of 'love'.

David: That's true, you could say just the same thing about 'love', because that is inside you and hard to communicate. Perhaps the words are there, but they are not words which are used very much. If somebody is in love then they want to tell the world about it because it makes them feel good. Whereas if you've got pain it's not something you want to write poetry about or tell the world. Some people do, that's true, but I mean how many pop songs are about love, and how many about having pain or being ill?

Chairman: All of them, by the sound of the modern ones!

[*Wild laughter and protest.*]

Liz: Yes, most of the pop songs around seem to be about the problem of being in love.

Robert: If you wrote a song about the boil on your big toe I don't think that it would necessarily make the charts.

Chairman: It would hardly be a toe-tapper. Is this passage making a valid medical point?

Stuart: Yes, it is.

Tony: It makes an important point about language: the fact that there are no common folk terms with which you can express pain in a way that will be understood by everyone. Our language seems to be preoccupied with thought, concepts, and reason, rather than with feelings such as pain, suffering, or anguish.

David: And pain is something where you do need to tell the doctor whether it's colicky, or whether it radiates, and what its nature is; whereas with love there is no strict need to describe it to anybody else–particularly the exact sensation of it.

Gillian: There very well might be!

Chairman: David, one could say that the whole of love poetry is an attempt to articulate the experience of love.

David: Yes, but there's not the same urgency or need about it as there would be for the patient explaining his symptoms to a doctor.

Liz: I disagree with that. If I could just say something which really isn't relevant to medicine: I believe there may be just such an urgency for an individual to express his feelings of love, and it might be just as frustrating for him not to be able to as a patient who can't tell a doctor about a symptom.

Rod: I don't think all those love poems, and all that sort of thing, can ever state the exact feelings which a person is trying to convey.

Tony: On Rod's point, I don't think that even T. S. Eliot believed there had to be fidelity between the poet and the transfer of what the poet is saying to the reader. The person who reads the poem may construct their own meaning of it, and that interpretation may be as valid as the poet's.

Rod: Could I come back to give an answer to Tony. If you're talking about love and you're trying to convey that feeling to another person, it doesn't really matter whether or not they get the same feeling as you had. But when you're talking about pain, the patient will say something and he's got a feeling of what he means. The doctor must get the same feeling if there's going to be meaningful communication.

Chairman: I agree Rod. I think one of the most unsatisfactory questions for a student in his early clinical years to ask a patient is, 'What's the pain like?'

Hilary: Yes I agree, they say, 'Oh doctor, I can't tell you that'.

Robert: The answer frequently given is, 'Well, it's just a pain!' or 'Well what do you mean, what's it like?'

Hilary: David was describing an urgent personal need to describe the pain, well I think a lot of patients can't see the need to pinpoint the character of a pain in the way the doctor wants them to. To them the pain is just there and awful, and they think, 'Why should I have to explain it in detail?' Under those circumstances the patient can't see that it will be an advantage to them in helping the doctor find out what's wrong with them. The patient just doesn't think about the pain in the same diagnostic way as the doctor does.

Brendan: Another point in relation to the inability to articulate pain is that the first time anyone does it is when they've got a pain. Now while many other human feelings are talked about in the abstract, that isn't the case with pain. I also agree with what Hilary says, that once a patient has a pain and has told the doctor they've got it, they think that's enough. They expect that he should be able to make the diagnosis on their description because that's all they've experienced.

Robert: I think the sensation of pain tends to be forgotten as soon as it is past.

Gillian: That would depend on how bad it was. I think patients who have severe pains remember them vividly. Is there a difference between the significance that a word has for a person and the actual common meaning of it?

Chairman: Well that certainly is an important point in a clinical context, or at least in the context of communication. As Rod suggests, verbal communication surely depends on common understanding or mutual agreement of what a word means.

In a medical interview we have certain advantages. Unlike the situation at a cocktail party or a social gathering, we don't have to face many of the ambiguities and deceits of normal social play. A patient doesn't usually come to try and deceive his doctor. The patient may not be completely open with the doctor for reasons of fear, shame, or (very occasionally) malingering. But most commonly patients are honest with their doctors. Their basic premise is trust. But then we come to the problems of 'words'. Some words have a common meaning, but others have meanings which will vary with an individual's life experience of the word, or the concept which the word implies. Let's consider my comment in relation to James Joyce's passage from *A Portrait of the Artist as a Young Man:* young Stephen Dedalus is talking to a priest.

> The language in which we are speaking is his before it is mine. How different are the words *home*, *Christ*, *ale*, *master*, on his lips and on mine! I cannot speak or write these words without unrest of spirit. His language, so familiar and so foreign, will always be for me an acquired speech. I have not made or accepted its words. My voice holds them at bay. My soul frets in the shadow of his language.[6]

Colin: The passage seems to be making the point that a person who is listening to somebody else, may *hear* what the person is trying to say but can't actually *appreciate* the personal significance of what they're saying.

Stuart: I think there's a professional message for us in this passage. It's not a doctor here, it's a priest. When a priest speaks, it does tend to produce a certain amount of reverence. A priest does seem to say things slightly differently. It must be similar for some people when a doctor speaks. Even listening to different medical colleagues making a similar comment, it sometimes sounds very different.

Tony: James Joyce may have been making a broader point than just a difference in word meaning and the associated problem of understanding language between two people. He was also concerned with the deficiencies in the form of language. I mean, if you compare some of his earlier works with what he did in Molly Bloom's dream scene in *Ulysses*, it's just incredible the way he uses language there. It was almost like a vomiting of his mind onto the paper.

Chairman [*laughing*]: Tony, some people call that 'genius'. Could we go on from what Colin was saying about the importance of understanding what a word means to a patient, to a question of how we can exploit that particular meaning in our communication with that patient–especially when we are trying to explain something? In other words, can we put our explanation in the patient's words rather than our own? Can anyone give me any examples of this?

Rod: Well, if you're talking to children you could simplify your language and use their vocabulary and concepts rather than adult ones.

Robert: If you were talking to a simple patient you would have to use short sentences and very simple words. It really doesn't matter who it is, all patients will be different and you have to tune in to each individual patient. Your technique of interview has to be modified with almost every consultation.

Chairman: Can the use of metaphor help when describing things to patients?

Rod: Yes it can, for example if you were describing urinary problems to a patient you might use a plumbing metaphor.

Colin: If you were explaining to somebody that they had heart failure, and they had mechanical knowledge, you might use the analogy of a fuel pump.

Chairman: If a tradesman had atherosclerosis you might explain the disease in terms of rusting of pipes, to relate decreased blood flow and decreased water flow.

Gillian: Yes.

Tony: I remember a doctor telling a story about a patient who thought the concept of a blocked tube meant that he was gradually blowing up, and blowing up, and blowing up, and that if he kept drinking he would finish up bursting. Now that might be O.K. for a patient with acute retention, but I don't think it's a helpful concept for one who has congestive heart failure.

Liz: A handy analogy for patients who have conditions which are just due to wear and tear (arthritis and things like that), is to use the wearing out of a motor car in the explanation. I think the fact that you can't replace parts, especially if the models are out of date, gets the message across.

Hilary: One approach, when you're trying to explain to the patient what his disease is like, is to ask him to explain to you (as the doctor), what he understands the condition to mean. Then you can work on that. That would help to eliminate misunderstanding.

Chairman: Good; in other weeks we have discussed fear and ignorance as hindrances to communication, so perhaps we won't go over them again today. We have just considered the problem of word meaning and word use. Now let's move on to another dimension of the communication task: the non-verbal. Let's do this by reading a passage from D. H. Lawrence's novel, *Sons and Lovers*.

> Sometimes he came in, very pale and still, with watchful, sudden eyes, like a man who is drunk almost to death. They were both afraid of the veils that were ripping between them.
>
> Then she pretended to be better, chattered to him gaily, made a great fuss over some scraps of news. For they had both come to the condition when they had to make much of the trifles, lest they should give in to the big thing, and their human independence would go smash. They were afraid so they made light of things and were gay. Sometimes as she lay he knew she was thinking of the past. Her mouth gradually shut hard in a line. She was holding herself rigid, so that she might die without ever uttering the great cry that was tearing from her. He never forgot that hard, utterly lonely and stubborn clenching of her mouth, which persisted for weeks.[7]

Nicholas: I think this is a very moving passage. What we are being shown is two people sharing a common tragedy. In this case they're not externalizing it; they're not expressing it.

Hilary: Yes, they're purposefully avoiding any expression which would force them to confront what is going on.

Robert: I agree they're internalizing it, but I don't agree that it's not being expressed. I mean there's a tremendous amount of non-verbal expression here. He had 'watchful sudden eyes, like a man who is drunk almost to death.' There would be no mistaking that expression.

Colin: They're trying to internalize it so much that they're probably expressing their feelings much more than if they engaged in open talk.

Chairman: Yes; we were discussing that point last week when Hilary commented that Lady Muriel's request to 'watch every word' would create such an artificial state that it would be more embarrassing to the Master than open speech. What's the message in this passage for us as doctors in relation to non-verbal communication?

Rod: Frequently we see a patient who chatters gaily about something, who seizes on all sorts of scraps of news and incidents, and beneath it all is quite a worry.

Brendan: As doctors, we also use the unspoken aspects of communication.

Liz: I think 'unspoken' contact between a doctor and patient is absolutely vital to clinical communication. We are not as conscious of its presence as we should be, and that's a pity because there is so much potential understanding that the doctor can pick up through an awareness of gestures.

Colin: It's frequently in this area that much care and consideration is expressed between people, because it's not the things said, it's the things shown which are important.

Brendan: Quite often, when you're on a ward round and dealing with a terminal patient, you can't really say very much which is meaningful. The people and the doctors who I have observed and admire in that situation are those who are reassuring, and concerned, and receptive, without hardly saying a word. In that situation I think you have to be aware when the patient wants some privacy.

Jane: But a very close relationship with your patients is needed to reduce the chance of them misinterpreting your actions and unspoken gestures.

Chairman: What about touching the patient?

Gillian: I think touching is very important because it helps the patient feel they can talk to you, and that you're listening to them.

Colin: Touching the patient relaxes them, they don't shuffle around the bed, and they don't feel they've got to avoid you. Just holding somebody's hand, whether or not you're taking their pulse, can reassure them. I think holding a patient tends to calm them down.

Chairman: I agree with you. I am a great believer in some sort of physical contact with the patient. One almost feels there is an energy which moves between you at the point of contact.

David: We are in a very fortunate position in the medical profession because there aren't the barriers to touching another human being which there are according to normal social conventions. I think it would be difficult for a lawyer to walk up to a client and touch them in the way that we can.

Chairman: I think that's true too. One can embrace a distressed patient in the ward or in a clinic without any amorous connotation being put on it by an observer, the patient, or yourself.

Liz: I agree with what you've said. When you touch a patient they understand that, at that moment, you are committed to them and that you're paying attention to what is going on from their point of view.

Gillian: Touching a patient is a very hard thing for a student to do at first. I suppose it depends on the way you have been brought up, but touching another person is difficult for some people. I find it difficult. I don't know, perhaps it was the way I was brought up. Now I'm getting used to it, but earlier on I didn't find it at all easy to touch a patient.

Stuart: No one is suggesting it's easy!

Rod: Doesn't meaningful communication also mean that if you're talking to an old lady who is sitting in a chair, or a child, that you get down and talk to them at their level rather than stand above them.

Chairman: You have outlined the advantages of non-verbal communication but what about the disadvantages? In an earlier week Gillian suggested that if the doctor was performing in a way that was short of complete commitment, the patient could usually see straight through the shallowness. The doctor can't fool the patient if his gestures betray indifference.

Stuart: I agree it can work the other way, but it's not always that simple. If you've had a bad day, if you're tired, if you're worried about another patient (or for a multitude of different reasons), the distractions in your mind may be expressed in your face or behaviour, and the patient might easily draw the wrong conclusion that you're not interested.

Chairman: That's an important point, Stuart.

Continuing on this problem of unspoken communication and how subtle it can be, let's read a passage from Henry James's novel, *The Wings of the Dove*. It's not an easy passage, and I have shortened it to try to make it easier to read. The context of the passage is that a doctor asks a patient, 'Do you have any relatives?' What follows is a communication between them during which no word is spoken. What we are given is really a revelation of what is going on in the girl's mind.

> Wanting to know more about a patient than how a patient was constructed or deranged couldn't be, even on the part of the greatest doctors, anything but some form or other of the desire to let the patient down easily. When that was the case the reason, in turn, could only be, too manifestly, pity; and when pity held up its tell-tale face like a head on a pike, in a French revolution, bobbing before a window, what was the inference but that the patient was bad? He might say what he would now—she would always have seen the head at the window; and in fact from this moment she only wanted him to say what he would. . . . if he was making her talk she was talking; and what it could, at any rate, come to for him was that she wasn't afraid. . . . there actually passed between them for some seconds a sign, a sign of the eyes only, that they knew together where they were. This made, in their brown old temple of truth, its

> momentary flicker; then what followed it was that he had her, all the same, in his pocket; and the whole thing wound up, for that consummation, with its kind dim smile. . . . 'Do you mean,' he asked, 'that you've no relations at all?—not a parent, not a sister, not even a cousin nor an aunt?'[8]

Chairman: I don't think this is an easy passage. What do you feel it's saying?

David: It starts off by saying that when a doctor tries to find out more than a patient feels is necessary for the diagnosis and management of their condition, he will make them feel uneasy. The patient might conclude that the reason you're probing them is that they have something badly wrong with them and you want to let them down easily.

Rod: All through life most people have had a special relationship with their parents or guardians: parents sign forms for you, take you to school—everything is deferred to one's parents. They are also there to help you when things go wrong. I think the actual question asked here is of special importance, because when the doctor asks 'Don't you have any relatives?' one can see how the girl would automatically think, 'Maybe I'm going to die', 'Maybe they are going to need the relatives to tidy up my affairs', or 'Maybe I'm going to need relatives to support me as I get sicker.'

Colin: In a way, this doctor could be using the question as a feeler, as if to say, 'Do you want me to tell you what is going on?' I think she's more or less answered: when it says, 'there actually passed between them for some seconds a sign, a sign of the eyes only, that they knew together where they were.' The communication seems to me to have been answered, and then they go on.

Chairman: And what did she communicate to him?

Colin: I think she communicated that she wasn't afraid and that she would like to know just as much as he wanted to tell her.

Gillian: Don't you find that often when you start asking a patient about their job, or what they like doing with themselves in their spare time, that they suddenly start to get scared? As soon as you take yourself away from purely clinical things, they sometimes back up.

Chairman: That does happen occasionally. Are there any particular groups of patients who may get a little bit suspicious with the feeling that they were under an inquisition?

Colin: I think motor-car accident cases might, particularly if they felt they were culpable.

Gillian: Men sometimes feel uneasy, especially if a female doctor is asking them questions.

Brendan: Patients who are in the transitional zone between organic illness and psychological illness frequently dislike being cross-examined intensely.

Colin: I think young people, more so than old, dislike that sort of approach.

Chairman: What about the simpler sort of person; or the person who is economically under-privileged. Do they like the close questioning of the medical interview?

Liz: It's professional people and intelligent people who dislike close questioning.

Brendan: Most of the less intelligent patients whom I have spoken to are quite ready to answer the questions, they are among the most trusting of patients.

[*General agreement.*]

Gillian: Yes, they frequently appreciate the concern of someone who they feel is more intelligent than them.

David: The thing that worries me about asking a patient what their job is, is that when they say, 'Oh, I'm a labourer' or 'a working man on the roads' I don't know what to say. I mean what does one say then? You can't say, 'Oh, that's smashing.' As a doctor how do you relate to a vocational experience which is totally strange to you?

Chairman: That's a good question. How do doctors confront the socio-economic gap which may exist between them and their patients?

Gillian: You can say, 'How long have you been doing it,' and 'Do you like it?', and so on.

David: Yes I know that, but I just find it so hard not to be condescending in that situation.

Many students [*trying to speak together*].

Chairman: Just a moment, David is making an important point, he is saying that it's an uneasy moment in the interview when you feel that the patient is feeling just a little bit patronized by your question.

David: Maybe I'm just paranoid about giving that impression, but it does worry me.

Nicholas: And you can take the other side of the equation: the doctor himself might start to feel insecure and uneasy in that situation.

Hilary: I think the problem often arises with women who aren't working. When you ask such a patient, 'What do you do?' they are forced into saying, 'Oh, I'm just a housewife.' They are made to feel they're doing nothing.

Liz: But you can get over that by saying, 'Oh, I suppose you enjoy the children', or something like that.

Hilary: I still don't think it's as easy as a man who can say, 'I do such and such.' Women have a sense of vocational emptiness.

Liz: The same could be said about a man who is out of work, or who has been made redundant. Don't you feel sometimes that when a patient says, 'I'm a labourer' that you're embarrassed because you feel the patient is aware of the discrepancy between your vocation and his? It's difficult not to create the impression that you're a young medical student on the way up, and they are a nobody.

Nicholas: In part, the doctor is responsible for the impression he creates. I think if you are being genuine and not asking the question in a murmur as though you shouldn't be asking it–if you are not making it anything special–the patient will look at it differently. You are not giving the patient a tick or a cross on the basis of their answer to that question. He shouldn't be made to feel ashamed.

Liz: Yes, but don't you think that some patients feel that you *are* giving them a tick or a cross when you ask them what their job is or how they spend their time. That's the feeling I get from some patients; it's as though they're aware of my judgement on their job or style of life.

Brendan: If you approach this question as routinely as any other question in the medical history, you can avoid this sort of embarrassment. I don't see it as a big problem. I think you can get over it very easily by going on to the next question, 'How many children do you have?', 'Are you married?', and so on.

Gillian: I think that's just brushing the problem aside.

Many students [*trying to speak together.*]

Chairman: Occasionally, what a man does is important to his medical condition. I mean in the case of a labourer you could ask him, 'What safety precautions are taken on the job?, 'Is he exposed to noise or chemicals?', and things like that.

Tony: But there are other aspects besides the purely medical significance of the question, 'What do you do for a living?' I think it is sad that the question can take on such enormous significance. It seems bad that we are so preoccupied with these status questions and feelings of superiority and condescension toward the patient.

Gillian: But it worries the patient though!

Chairman: Tony, I believe that if these feelings of difficulty exist for doctors then we should discuss them.

Tony: I'm not trying to run away from them, but I'm not trying to laud them either. I think they exist, I feel them too, but I think it's sad.

Gillian: That doesn't mean we should dismiss them.

Stuart: I think the main thing is for the doctor to show a genuine interest in the patients and in the questions he's asking them.

Gillian: But what's genuine? What is genuine to you maybe misinterpreted or misunderstood by the patient.

Stuart: No. If I meet a patient for the first time and ask them what they do, and they say, 'I work on the roads', I don't find that boring or embarrassing. I don't say, 'Oh, you work on the roads.'

Brendan: It's a function of the doctor, not the patient. If your attitude is one which shows some understanding, and you don't attach any great socio-economic significance to the patient's job or attitudes, then there's no uneasiness at all.

Rod: Brendan said it's not a function of the patient, it's a function of the doctor. Well I think it's a function of both. There are doctors who react to it and there are patients who do as well.

Tony: What I'm saying is that when patients say to you I'm a labourer or a boot-polisher, I think it's a bit of a presumption for a doctor automatically to feel that they're dreadfully ashamed of who they are and what they do.

Gillian: No; we are not saying that—we're talking about the specific examples where the patient *does* feel ashamed or the doctor *does* feel embarrassed.

David: I agree with Gillian. I'm not saying by any means that a majority of patients feel like this, but one does get the impression that some are ashamed to tell you what they do. You can't just gloss over the patient's embarrassment and say 'Yes.' It's just like when you ask a patient, 'Are you married?' and she replies with, 'I was, but my husband died three years ago, thank God. He was a real bastard!' Now you can't avoid making a response; you can't run away from it; the patient is almost challenging you for a response when they say something like that.

Tony: Yes, that's true.

David: Sometimes a patient seems to want to say something about some aspect of their life which we might assume as being embarrassing to them, but which they seem perfectly open about. They want to talk about it.

Nicholas: And what would you gain by saying something to the patient at that point?

Gillian, Rod and David [*all trying to speak together*]: Well, it depends on what the patient really wants, they might welcome an opportunity to talk.

Jane: I think you should always let the patient speak about whatever they want to, but we don't have the right to pass judgements on what they have said to us.

Colin: I agree. I think if a patient throws out any sign a doctor has got to take it up, no matter what it is.

Liz: Coming back to the passage, I think the importance of asking a question like 'Do you have any relatives?' will vary with when you ask it. If you do it naturally in the early part of the history, when you are asking the personal details of marriage and where the patient lives and so on, it falls naturally into place and the patient doesn't get upset about it. But if it is asked after you have received the result of a special test, or after you have made an examination, or after the patient had been seen by a specialist, that might cause distress.

Chairman: When you ask a question *is* important. For example, when you ask a mother the family history, and ask her about the health of her children, her response is occasionally a fear that her condition may be contagious to her children, or that it may be hereditary.

Jane: In this passage, obviously the way the doctor has asked the question 'Have you any relatives?' has been bad, because the patient indicates she is not going to believe anything he tells her now. She says, 'He might say what he would now–she would always have seen the head at the window'. It implies that he has had his turn to tell the truth and he's lost it.

Liz: I agree with Jane.

Rod: I don't think the patient is saying that.

Chairman: I'm surprised you say that Jane. I think one of the beauties of this passage is that, although verbal communication stops, a very subtle communication of the eyes takes place, and the communication continues.

Gillian: I agree. There is a communication which goes on between them. It says, 'there actually passed between them for some seconds a sign, a sign of the eyes only, that they knew together where they were.'

Jane: Well how do you explain the line, 'He might say what he would now–she would always have seen the head at the window'?

Chairman: I think that's the patient expressing her feeling that she understood perfectly why he was asking the question 'Do you have any relatives?' She realizes there is a very great possibility that she is gravely ill. But she then goes on to say that, having seen the doctor's gesture, she can't now be fooled. The important point is the one that follows: she conveys the feeling, 'I know what's in your mind, doctor and I'm not afraid of it.' He picks up her feeling and it's at that moment that they 'knew together where they were'.

Gillian: Yes; she has seen that there's pity there and she's responded.

Jane: Well what does the phase 'He might say what he would now' mean?

Chairman: I think what's being suggested there is that the doctor could say whatever he liked now, and it wouldn't matter, she would understand his real meaning.

Jane: Well that's the point I'm trying to make! She is considering the possibility that he may not tell the truth to her.

Chairman: I understand; but I think that the communication context of this passage is that he doesn't lie because he picks up a signal from her. That's the point that I hope the passage can bring out.

Jane: What about her feeling that 'he had her in his pocket, the whole thing wound up'?

Nicholas: I think the passage could be interpreted another way: that the doctor has made a value judgement on the significance of the disease for the patient, and now, in a sort of condescending way, he's going on with it. I agree that you could read it the way the chairman suggested, but I still think this is bad communication between the patient and the doctor.

Gillian: I don't think so. I don't think a doctor has to spell everything out. I think there has been a very delicate communication between them.

Jane: You still haven't answered my question about the doctor having the whole thing wound up, with the patient 'in his pocket'. I get the feeling from reading this passage that the doctor didn't intend to convey to the patient that she was seriously ill, but that he let it slip. It's only because the patient was sensitive that he was confronted with his error of communication.

Nicholas: Would this be the sort of doctor who would elicit the meaning and significance of what's going on from the patient's point of view? I mean there is something really rather profound going on for the patient here.

Gillian: I think you've got to allow the patient the capacity of understanding certain signs and gestures without always spelling it out with words. It's up to the doctor to work out how much the patient understands. It will vary with their appreciations and intelligence. I don't think it all has to be done in words at all.

Jane: I'm not saying that this patient hasn't understood, what I am saying is that the patient *has* understood, but perhaps the doctor didn't mean the patient to understand as much as she has, and he's been forced into conceding something.

Chairman: But you would agree Jane, that having let it slip, a communication between them did continue from that point?

Rod: I don't think he did let it slip accidentally, because there is a line which says that 'they knew together where they were'.

Chairman: I don't necessarily agree with that Rod—I mean he could have let it slip and then in the communication which followed they mutually understood the meaning and the implication of the slip.

I don't think this passage is a particularly easy one so I haven't tried to limit the discussion. I put it in to add a final dimension to the span of communication that we have been considering today: starting with a consideration of the confusion that can arise with the use of technical medical words, together with the confusion that comes through the use of a common word in a medical context; moving on to words which we all use but which have different meanings to different people, added to which are the unspoken communication gestures which are obvious, and finally to the very subtle gestures that are picked up by perceptive patients—we can appreciate the complexity of communication problems. And we haven't even considered the problem of patients who can't speak the language. For some of them the problems are frightening.

Now I want to come back to something Stuart said earlier when he suggested that communication can break down for a whole number of reasons, some of which I think he mentioned: the doctor may be tired, or may be upset, and so on. I would like to go round the group and ask your opinion about what sort of things impair the ideal clinical communication.

Brendan: A lack of commitment, on the part of the doctor, to what is going on is important.

Nicholas: A lack of personal equality between the patient and the doctor. This can be educational, it can be class, it can be economic, it can be sex or age—anything where, from any point of view, a patient is different from the doctor. Each will hinder the communication and will require greater effort.

Gillian: As you said before, I think foreign patients or patients from a different cultural background have remarkable problems.

Liz: Differences in intelligence between the patient and the doctor: I think the simple patient needs special consideration.

Robert: If the doctor has something going on in his personal life, some upheaval or worry, if he's not getting on with his wife, if he's unhappy, if his children are unwell, if he's worried about promotion in his job, or worried about any number of personal problems, he may not be able to concentrate on his patient.

David: If the doctor is tired, if things aren't going well in the ward, or if a patient has got complications, it makes the communication more difficult.

Chairman: I agree, I think all doctors have been in the position of having a number of patients who aren't going as well as they should be, either as a result of the underlying condition or the doctor's treatment, and his confidence is undermined. When a doctor's confidence is gone, he doesn't feel like talking or communicating in the way he normally does.

Hilary: The actual physical conditions of the interview are important. Down in Outpatients where a patient has got only a bit of curtain around them and about twenty other people can listen in to what is being said, there's no privacy, and I don't think patients feel happy speaking, especially on the more personal or delicate issues.

Stuart: The stature of the medical profession as a whole can be a hindrance to some patients—just that fear and feeling that the doctor's got a sense of knowledge and power about what is going on while the patient is ignorant.

Tony: Lack of understanding of the deeper nature of the patient makes communication difficult.

Liz: Going back to what we were saying before, if the patient is embarrassed or frightened about anything then communication won't work. And as Brendan said last week, many patients only hear what they want to hear, no matter what you tell them.

Rod: If a patient has upset the doctor (just as Septimus upset Bradshaw) and the doctor takes a dislike to the patient, or the other way around, if the patient takes a dislike to the doctor, then the contact quickly deteriorates.

Chairman: And we have to remember that when a doctor is concentrating on what the patient is saying, he or she is frequently trying to write it all down at the same time.

Gillian: It's very important, even when you're writing, to look at the patient when you're talking to them. If you don't look they feel you're not listening.

Stuart: It's not possible to look at all patients because they talk so much and so fast that you can't write it all down and continue to look at them.

Chairman: But Gillian has made the point that eye contact is important in a consultation. Do you agree?

[*General comment*] Yes.

Chairman: Well what about when you're using an interpreter?

Gillian: It's pretty hard then, but it's still very important. In fact it's probably more important because you have to indicate to the patient that you're understanding what they are saying to the interpreter. It's much harder because there's another person in the way but . . .

Chairman: So you would be making more of an effort to look at a patient rather than the interpreter?

Gillian: Yes, I would.

Chairman: I think that's a very important point, and so difficult to do.

Gillian: It's because you don't think. You're asking all the questions of the interpreter and you are getting all the answers back from them, it's very easy to ignore the patient.

Chairman: One of the areas I found difficult as a student was discussing a patient's sexual history. We haven't at any stage in this course discussed sexuality in relation to our patients and any problems in that area. Are there any problems?

Rod: Yes; I think there are. I think the first time a young doctor goes to examine a female patient, particularly a young female patient, he's under a lot of tension. The same applies when a young woman doctor goes to examine male patients. There's embarrassment on both sides.

Liz: Especially when you are examining older guys . . .

David: I saw a foreign patient from somewhere in the south of Europe who refused to be examined by a young woman doctor.

Gillian: If you feel any sexual attraction towards a patient, you have to ignore it completely.

Robert: Come on!

Gillian: I'm not saying it's a problem [*laughter*] but it's required of us that we've got to be completely bland, that we have to look upon patients as neutral objects, at least sexually.

Jane: It only becomes a problem if the doctor is embarrassed and he or she conveys that embarrassment to the patient. I suppose some doctors could try and compensate for the sexual interest that they may have by appearing to be distant and severe. And that makes it very unpleasant for the patient.

Liz: I think it's more of a problem for the patient. Patients are frequently more embarrassed than we are, especially the patient who isn't sure of our attitude of neutrality.

Brendan: I would like to agree with Liz. For the most part doctors handle it satisfactorily, it is just one of many things a doctor has to ignore as part of the role which is expected of him. But I think a lot of patients do get embarrassed because it's a new experience for *them*.

Chairman: Which sort of patients may be embarrassed by the sexuality of a clinical situation—the physical exposure for example?

Liz: I think little old ladies do. Especially if they've never been married.

Robert: Teenage girls are sometimes distressed by physical examination.

Rod: And teenage boys also.

Stuart: I agree, and I think teenage boys feel embarrassment a little earlier than teenage girls. Most young boys seem to be more self-conscious than girls at a very early age in puberty.

Chairman: Puberty can be a hair-raising experience.

[*Wild laughter.*]

Colin: I think problems can arise with the long-term patient. I mean, if you are looking after a patient for a long time and you are committed to them, then I think very close feelings can develop, and mutual attraction can follow.

Chairman: How do you handle the situation when a patient becomes interested in the doctor, I mean interested sexually?

Stuart: A cold shower?

[*Laughter.*]

David: Well I suppose it depends just what the patient looks like!

[*Wild laughter.*]

Chairman: I remember this once happened to me when I was a student doing psychiatry. During one of the interviews the patient confessed to the consultant psychiatrist that she was sexually attracted to me. When he asked her why, she said because 'He looks like an intellectualized version of Elvis Presley'!

[*Laughter.*]

Chairman: How confident do you feel about asking patients their sexual history?

Liz: This is a problem area.

Gillian: Yes, I think because we're embarrassed it becomes a problem area.

Hilary: It depends most on whether or not the patient feels it is relevant to their medical problem. If a patient comes in with something which they feel is completely unrelated to their sexual life, then I think they get embarrassed and wonder what's going on.

Chairman: And yet if a patient comes in with an ingrowing toenail, we still, in the course of a full history, take gastro-intestinal, urinary, and cardio-respiratory system details—why is sexual history excluded from this?

Tony: That's not quite the same thing. After all, we don't run around doing things to each other in terms of our gastro-intestinal function. One has the fear that the patient will think that one's becoming voyeuristic if one is probing into areas which don't immediately seem relevant. Most patients don't like people intruding into their personal life and doctors are not excluded from that.

David: We get taught a hell of a lot about gastro-intestinal function, but we get taught damn all about sexual function. That's one area where our expertise is not assured.

Liz: And so in that way we don't feel confident if a patient does come to us with any sexual problems.

Chairman: So you seem to have identified two areas: one, a defect in a doctor's education, and the other, patient embarrassment. Together they are not conducive to a good medical communication on sexual matters.

Hilary: That's specially true if you are talking to a 40-year-old male or female and you're only a 21-year-old medical student. They're almost certainly going to think, 'How can this young person have any more experience or understanding than what I've got?', and, 'How can they help me?' And that may be true.

Stuart: I disagree. It's the same problem as whether or not a doctor needs to have experienced a disease or a condition in order to have some understanding of it. I mean, we don't all think we have to experience appendicitis to be able to understand what is going on in a patient who has appendicitis. Why is sexual activity any different? Why is sexual experience necessary for understanding the sexual aspects of patient care?

Colin: I'd like to take Stuart up on that, I think. Sexual problems are so concerned with the problems of living that I wouldn't underestimate the importance of some experience in helping the doctor to understand the patient. On sexual matters experience counts for much more than it does on a straight medical exercise like the treatment or diagnosis of appendicitis.

Liz: Are you saying because it's more psychological rather than organic, that it's . . .

Colin: No. I just think you need some experience to deal well with sexual problems. I think it takes time to build up an appreciation of sexual problems. It's not gained from just going to books and reading up about it in the way that you can get a reasonably adequate knowledge of a medical condition.

Liz: I'm still not clear why you're making a distinction between the need for a doctor to have experienced sexuality in order to understand it, but not necessarily having the need to experience diseases in order to understand them.

Colin: Well I tried to explain. In Stuart's example of appendicitis, you can go and look it up in a book. But which books have you used to look up sexual problems? You must rely on experience to some extent.

Tony: I think that this reinforces David's earlier point that there is no way that you can get adequate coverage of those topics in a medical book. The questions are too complex for a textbook. Sexual preferences are so variable.

Liz: As I understand it Colin's talking about the doctor's personal experience in sex.

Colin: Yes I am.

Liz: Then I don't understand.

Stuart: No, neither do I.

Colin: It's not just the personal experience of specific sex, but relating that to the whole area of problems of living and how sex can affect life in general. Now that's not easy to get from a book. I don't think it's easy to appreciate a sexual matter from the patient's point of view. It's not something that can be formally learnt.

Stuart: I just want to make the point that I was making an analogy between appendicitis and sexual *experience*, not the technical aspect. What I am trying to say is that, in part, if you are talking to a 50-year-old who you are sure has had an experience which you haven't had, then that's not all that much different from speaking to a patient who has had appendicitis, an experience you might not have had either.

Chairman: Stuart is saying that, when a doctor deals with a medical condition that he hasn't experienced himself, he has to use some degree of human imagination to appreciate what it means for the patient, and that it is the same with sexual problems. However, Colin is saying that as sexual activity is more of a common denominator to us all, and as it is related to human relationships in general, it is unlike appendicitis or perforated peptic ulcer, and therefore experience would obviously be an advantage.

Gillian: You're assuming a lot by saying that!

[*Laughter.*]

Chairman: I agree there are differences in sexual preference and in sexual techniques, but I think there is some truth in Colin's point. The likelihood of shared common experience through personal experience is more probable in dealing with sexual matters than with purely medical problems–and might be more important.

Liz: If you've got a young guy who's a homosexual, or a young unmarried mother who comes in with guilt feelings then I think it is a matter of experience to some extent. But obviously the same doctor couldn't have experienced both.

David: Colin was saying just before that it's not just a matter of technique. Most sexual problems which present are problems of human relationships. I agree, I think they're related much more to problems of human relationships than they are to purely technical aspects of sex . . .

Colin: And that's why some human experience on the part of the doctor is so necessary to deal with them . . .

David: And Gillian was implying that maybe everyone isn't sexually experienced. But everyone has had common human relationships–and it is those human relationships which are basic to understanding sexual problems. Most people don't suffer from their lack of specific sexual experience in dealing with sexual problems.

Stuart: There are also different cultural and social taboos.

Chairman: What do you think the answer would be if you went down the street and asked one hundred people, 'If you had some problem in relation to sexuality would you feel as confident in talking to your doctor about it as you would a symptom in relation to a specific medical condition?'

Gillian: Usually 'No.'

Chairman: I'm ignorant as to what your formal medical course exposure has been on the problems and discussions in relation to sex. What have you had?

Liz: Zero.
Gillian: No; we had a few discussions last year.
David: I think any exposure is helpful.

[*Laughter.*]

Hilary: I don't think all the formal education in the world is going to make up for lack of your own experience.
Liz: But there are thousands of things we can't experience, but we have to know about them in being doctors.
Eight students [*trying to speak together.*]
Chairman: But don't you think, Hilary, that in discussions students can cross-fertilize each other? [*Wild laughter.*] Sorry, I didn't mean that.
Nicholas: I think there's another problem in relation to the difficulty of a male doctor understanding the specific sexual problems of a woman, and the opposite is true as well.
Liz: Oh no!
Chairman: Well Liz, you say 'no', but as a rule do you believe that women patients prefer to speak to women doctors about their sexual problems, or male doctors?
Liz: I think that depends on the female.
Colin: I don't.
Gillian: I think they'd rather speak to women doctors.
Rod: The fact that women go to see women doctors has nothing to do with the fact that men can't understand women's problems, it's because the females are embarrassed.
Tony: Surely that embarrassment is symptomatic of something deeper, perhaps it's a deficiency on the part of the male doctor or the society.
Brendan: One of the reasons women go to see women doctors is that they realize in every contact between male and female there is the potential for sexual interest. It may just be a matter of safety.
Chairman: As medical students, what is the most difficult area that you have found in relation to the sexual side of dealing with patients? [*Silence.*] Is it an area which you have skirted around when talking to patients?

[*General agreement*] Yes.

Chairman: Why?
Nicholas: I think because, to a large extent, sexual discussions depend on a good rapport with the patient, and everything about being a student subverts your ability to have such a relationship with the patient. Most of us as students feel frightened of imposing

ourselves on patients. That's especially so when we're in an area that isn't all that relevant to the management of the patient.

Liz: I think it's a deficiency in our education. I certainly don't feel confident about dealing with anyone's sexual problems.

Stuart: You feel inferior as a student too. You've got no responsibilities to the patient at all, no meaningful responsibilities. If you feel yourself that you are putting the patient through an embarrassing situation just for the hell of it, or for some theoretical reason, it's wrong. You're not the physician looking after them.

Brendan: Exactly the same problem comes up when you're doing rectal examinations on patients, and you're only doing them to 'learn'. You always feel uncomfortable that you are putting the patient through an ordeal that is of no benefit to them whatsoever.

Gillian: What about somebody who is impotent because they're on antihypertensive drugs? What do you say to a patient who asks you about that?

Chairman: That's opened up a whole new area in relation to sexual problems; the specific medical conditions or medical therapies which can affect sexual function. Now, how confident do you feel about those? For example you might have a patient who is going to have a radical mastectomy who asks you what effect it is going to have on her sex life. Or a man who is going to have an abdomino-perineal excision for cancer of the rectum, who is also worried about his sexual activity and ability to get an erection.

Gillian: That's right. I just wouldn't know what to say to those patients.

Chairman: Well *should* we know?

Liz: Yes we should. As students we should be taught this but it never comes up. It's appalling the lack of teaching on sexual matters.

David: I was annoyed a couple of nights ago. I was looking up the surgical textbook which is one of the prescribed texts for students in our university, and I was reading up about prostatectomies. One of the things I was interested in finding out was, what is the post-operative incidence of sexual problems. All the book said was that sterility occurs because ejaculation occurs into the bladder. And I thought 'well, big deal'. That's not the most important aspect of a man's sexual concern. It disappointed me considerably and I thought it was just symbolic of the general lack in our education. If I was going to have my prostate out one of the first things I would want to know is what effect it was going to have on my sexual function. As students we should be able to answer those questions.

Chairman: Well time is nearly up for this session and this discussion but I'm glad we had it because we must not run away from this problem of sexuality.

Gillian: Who's running!

ESSAY 5

THE ORNAMENT OF LEARNING

Tis education forms the common mind;
As the twig is bent so the tree's inclined.[1]
Alexander Pope

One of the points made by the students towards the end of our last session was that during the medical course there is usually very little consideration given to the role and responsibilities of medical students. They are expected to attend in a dutiful fashion, to apply themselves diligently, and to pass the examinations set.

All students are expected to work hard, in particular to work hard on the specific and narrow area of learning medical facts. This is a philosophy which would have appealed to Emile Zola, who, in a lecture given to a new intake of students, expressed the following sentiment:

> I am therefore going to finish by proposing to you a faith, and by beseeching you to have a faith in work. Work, young people! I well know how trivial such advice appears: no speech-day passes at which it is not reflected amid the general indifference of the scholars. But, I ask you to reflect on it . . . I have had but one faith, and one strength—work! What has sustained me was the enormous labour I set myself. Before me stood always in the distance the goal towards which I was marching, and when life's hardships had cast me down, that sufficed to set me on my feet and give me courage to advance in spite of all. The work of which I speak to you is the regular work, the daily task, the duty one has undertaken to advance one step each day towards fulfilment of one's engagement. . . .
>
> Work! Remember, gentlemen, that is the sole law of the world, the regulator bringing organic matter to its unknown goal! Life has no other meaning . . . It is true work solves no metaphysical problems; it is but an empiric recipe enabling one to live one's life honestly and more or less tranquilly; but is it a small thing to obtain a sound state of moral and physical health and to escape the dangers of dreams . . .?
>
> What a healthy and great society that will be—a society each member of which will bear his reasonable share of work! A man who works is always kind.[2]

And just what is this work we set most of our students? How worthwhile and how relevant is it? Should we be satisfied?

It seems to me that as medical educators we deceive ourselves. We proclaim certain ideals and expect students to strive after them while we neither measure nor reward them. We imply certain educational objectives but ignore them in teaching: objectives like being able to cope with clinical uncertainty, or being able to assess the multitude of factors which influence a diagnostic or therapeutic probability, or the ability to acknowledge the importance of the human factors in a clinical situation. We neither stimulate nor reward sensitivity in our students. Like Dickens' Mr Gradgrind we wallop our students with demands for facts, facts, and more facts.

We cannot expect students to take seriously those qualities which we profess are essential, yet which they see us dismiss, ignore, or violate. It is my opinion that more errors are committed in medical practice due to lack of care, lack of communication, lack of human sensitivity, or to a lack of understanding of human nature, than are ever caused by a lack of medical knowledge. The fault is ours. Our students receive little guidance on understanding basic human problems. They have very little demonstration of basic human communications, and virtually no discussion on the whole area of medical ethics. Their medical apprenticeship is served almost solely in the miasma of the major hospitals. Their course shrivels their range of sympathies.

If some of you think my censures unfair, let me confront you with a challenge. Ask any medical student who has completed the years of his or her medical school course some questions on the *facts* of medicine. They will be able to answer them with competence or excellence. My challenge is this: how many of them have been asked, at any time during their medical course, to explain something unexpected to a patient; to explain a diagnosis of cancer or a fatal prognosis; to talk to relatives about their fears or problems; to weigh up the special human considerations which influence a patient's decision to agree to an operation or his wish to go home; to assess the effect of hospitalization on a patient and his family; or to deal with an angry, irritated, or distressed patient. How many of them have been asked to write a letter to the patient's family doctor explaining the details of a case? And how many have paid visits into the homes of their patients? Time does not allow me to complete a list which is as expansive as it is damning of our fictional medical education.

And yet we continue. We persist in asking our students to study hard to learn facts and to pass exams.

And what of these exams? So much of a medical student's examination is the ceremonious use of words offered to the monarchs of learning who subject the student's mind to ritual probing. Medical teachers walk on verbal stilts and their authority as teachers acts as a hindrance to those who wish to learn. I know that there is a very considerable mass of medical fact which must be pressed into the student mind; but it is only the very soft mind which receives its impressions passively. Our educational colleagues are provoked to distraction by their need to grade students. They can hardly let a year go by without scratching their examination itch. If we are going to keep a grading system, I would rather see marks given for the questions students ask, and not just for the answers given to examiners' questions, for the former reveal not only what the student knows, but what he wants to know. They give a measure not of his static knowledge but his curiosity. They are the feature of his studentship which indicates the magnitude of his imaginative, intuitive and speculative faculties.

The problem is not just that medical school curricula do little to preserve and develop the student's imagination, but that the syllabus actually imperils it. The process of 'knowing' advances along a mental path beginning with something felt intuitively, then structured theoretically, and finally consolidated into a working truth by experiment or experience. Education in general, and medical education in particular, introduces the students somewhere between opinion and fact and directs them towards the latter. The whole conceptual, imaginative or intuitive area of thought is left neglected. Does the practical objective of medical education act as a damper on the richer aspects of student intellectual life?

I am not suggesting that imagination can be taught, but only that the delicate conditions which allow it to flourish should be cultivated and protected. For to make factual knowledge, which is the end point of an intellectual sequence, the ideal of that sequence, is like making senility the object of growth, or death the object of life. The most cherished gift is not the final proof, the confirmed reality, or the established fact; it is that rare element in the mind which first conceived its possibility–the imagination.

Some teachers regard medical education as the simple transfer of knowledge from those who have it, to those who have less: it is like an educative transfusion from a donor who has, to a recipient who hasn't. But what is happening to a student's intrinsic speculative haematopoiesis while this is going on? What does the marrow of a student's mind do when its idea corpuscles come from without? Do the natural leucocytes grow lazy and the platelets puny when the normal mind is transfused as though it had intellectual anaemia?

It is argued by some that it is through tutorials at the bedside that the teacher creates the conditions for the free flow of ideas; yet even there we find stasis of opinion and coagulation of thought. The constant streaming in of thoughts of others must confine and suppress our own. Then the student is but a willing follower of corporate opinion and common custom; and the profession already has an epidemic of such imaginatively impotent members.

Most medical examinations these days are of the short-answer sort. This movement towards yes-no answer alternatives in examination questions of the multiple-choice type has many advantages for both the examiner and the student. It probably measures what exams have always measured with some degree of accuracy. The revolution in favour of the multiple-choice exam question is almost complete. Carried forward by the forces of statistical significance, convenience, efficiency, speed, and fairness, it has successfully eliminated all elements of resistance. While one could concede that when constructed with imagination such exam papers can probe factual knowledge, and can test a candidate's ability to think a medical problem through while making decisions in sequence, one is left with a smouldering suspicion that such papers miss something. Perhaps the recognition that medicine is an art which deals with human beings.

I feel it to be true that this sort of exam, and the study habit it induces, reinforces a particular conditioning of thought: it stimulates a pattern of thinking based on exclusive alternatives. It reduces flexibility of thought and subtlety of thought. The student is forced to choose between midnight and midday; dusk and dawn do not exist. Nothing softens the bright glare of assumed truth, nor the gloom of absolute error. It creates an atmosphere of absolutism where–in actual medical practice–none exists.

Just as rustics who have neither clock nor calendar use a thousand successive tints and traits in a landscape to tell the time, so too doctors must use all their senses to assess the subtleties which contribute to a clinical decision. Medical decisions are not static, sterile things. They are always made against a temporal background in which a large number of variables are assessed and reassessed: early observations are compared with later ones to produce a flux of factors, all of which a doctor or student must consider. Such an intellectual discipline is not stimulated or searched for in the sort of examination which we set our students these days. For it, like most of medical training, does little to prepare a student for the grey zones which are so common in medical practice.

This is the tyranny of testing. We now teach only what it is possible to measure objectively. The examinations now dictate what is taught, rather than serve as a measure of how adequately we have achieved our original educational objectives.

Didactic teaching and examining of a problematic subject are alien to its nature and frustrate the sensitive student. By providing ready-made answers they absolve the student from the responsibility of striving for those processes of decision-making which are essential to fine doctorship or studentship. They produce paralysis of the intellectual apparatus, and cripple the flexibility of the mind. They create an artificial educational objective of *what is permitted*, or *what one needs to know for exams*. One of the fundamental objectives of my medical humanities course is to help to activate the intellectual, imaginative, and moral capacities of medical students without imposing a formula of *acceptable* or *approved* notions.

Let me put forward a few trial examination questions in an attempt to highlight what I believe is missing from our present fashion in medical exams. How do we feel our students would handle them?

> A 36-year-old woman who has been admitted for investigation of her anaemia receives word that the person who is looking after her children is not coping well. The patient asks to leave the ward to go home. Which factors would you consider in making your decision in relation to this request?
>
> A 41-year-old woman who has cancer of the breast, and on whom it is intended to perform a radical mastectomy, asks you what effect this will have on her sex life. What is your approach to the answer?
>
> A 38-year-old architect with three children is involved in a motor-car accident. Three months after admission, he is due to go home from a rehabilitation centre. His residual disabilities are a mildly altered personality, a slight speech defect, and some impairment of memory. What are the problems you anticipate for the patient; and which services would you recruit to help his future management?
>
> A 40-year-old businessman who is five days past an acute myocardial infarction (heart attack) tells you that he has been 'thinking about the way he has been living'. What do you think he means? How would you continue the conversation?
>
> A 34-year-old foreign mother of four children, who speaks poor English, develops a faecal fistula following what was thought to be an adequate resection and anastomosis of small bowel—performed for a strangulated femoral hernia. Her husband, who acts as her interpreter, is very agitated. How would you deal with the husband's concern?
>
> A 57-year-old man, who has a gastric ulcer which has characteristics strongly suspicious of malignancy, refuses your recommendation for an operation. What do you do?

I appreciate that some educational technologists would shy away from areas which are not 'scientific' or 'empiric'. They would claim that if a question cannot be recast in terms of facts, then the question is insoluble and probably unexaminable. They may go so far as to say the putting of such questions is unfair and unreal. They might even claim (in ignorance) that no one has the methods needed for the evaluation of such problems.

But I believe there is a difference between giving an answer to a question for which there is an 'answer' based on factual knowledge, and the ability to discuss both sides of a proposition for which there is no absolute answer. To say that such questions or propositions are 'unfair and unreal', or are in fact 'non-questions', is to deny all problematical questions. And to say that no one has the methods for evaluating such written material is to deny the existence of a whole examination structure which virtually all humanities faculties use to assess their students' written work. My proposition is a plea for the recognition that questions which involve human issues do not have easy yes-no answers. To say there is no value in asking students to consider the many facets of a complex and perhaps unanswerable problem is to bend one's knees a little too subserviently before the altar of science and educational technology.

While the acquisition of medical facts is an important part of medical apprenticeship, it is by no means the only significant medical task, and it certainly is not the most important human task. In an answer to Zola's address to the students, Leo Tolstoy gave this reply:

> It always seemed to me that only an irrational being, like the ant of the fable, could be excused for exalting work to the rank of a virtue and boasting of it. . . . the pride of work, makes not only ants but men cruel. Who does not know those men, inaccessible to truth or kindness, who are always so busy that they never have the time either to do good or even to ask themselves whether their work is not harmful?
>
> Work can no more be considered a virtue than nutrition. Work is a necessity, to be deprived of which involves suffering, and to raise it to the rank of a merit is as monstrous as it would be to do the same for nutrition . . .
>
> In my opinion, not only is work not a virtue, but in our ill-organized society it is often a moral anaesthetic like tobacco, wine, and other means of stupefying and blinding ourselves to the disorder and emptiness of our lives . . .
>
> So if I were called on to give one single piece of advice, the one I considered most useful for the men of our century, I should say this to them: 'For God's sake pause a moment, cease your work, look around you, think of what you are and what you ought to be—think of the ideal'.[3]

Putting aside the obvious piety in the old man's plea (for Tolstoy was nearly seventy when he wrote those words), I believe there is a message in this passage for medical students. The ideal of a medical apprenticeship is more than the ability to pass an examination. As medical educators we have a responsibility to pay more than lip-service to the ideals of a general medical education and a general cultural education, for both contribute to a student's humane understanding of human problems.

Before we rally our students with the call to work hard we should heed Tolstoy's warning. Hard work, like ambition, or loyalty, or solidarity, or commitment, is an ambiguous quality. It might be misdirected, it might be inappropriate, and, above all, it might be a substitute for the sort of personal stocktaking without which we quickly become fatigued human beings–cosy in the security of our habits and prejudice.

Teachers should encourage the students to keep the examination in a perspective which makes it appear distant and small. The ideal of studentship should not be the honours list alone.

Whatever the outcome of a student's exams (and this applies as much if it is excellent or average), it is not the arbiter of a successful studentship. Examination results are not an academic medal whose glint can blind from view all of those areas of a student's being which are lying ignored or dormant. They are no warrant of his talent for relating to people. They do not test his capacity for imaginative thinking. They are no measure of his sense of compassion.

Learning makes our tongues sharper, but not our hearts kinder.

SESSION 6

PUBLIC REGARD FOR PROFESSIONAL PERFORMANCE

Chairman: As this is both the last session of the course and your last teaching session of any kind for the whole year, I think we should keep it short, despite the importance of the topic, because I know you are all keen to get up to the pub.

In past weeks we have been considering our topics from the point of view of certain individuals: the patient, the patient's relatives, and the doctor. I thought we should conclude our course with a consideration of the concept of the profession as a whole. Let's start by considering what does the concept of 'a profession' imply?

[*Pause.*]

Brendan: It's a group of people basically involved with a similar vocational activity, bound together by a set of written and unwritten laws. It implies a number of moral responsibilities and certain ways of acting irrespective of specialist interests within that larger body. The behaviour desired of the profession is binding for all its members.

Dave: I think Brendan's hit right on it. When one thinks of the medical profession, as distinct from a particular trade which isn't necessarily bound by certain professional rules, one implies a code of professional behaviour.

Chairman: Are you saying that behaviour is expected of members of the medical profession which is not expected of plumbers, carpenters, actors, or dustmen?

Doug: They could have a different code, but the medical profession places a greater emphasis on trust and respect. One expects a good service from a plumber, that's his role. But for a doctor, because the nature of his work involves a much more intimate relationship with people, he is expected to behave in ways which will win respect.

Chairman: Doug, you've added a dimension to Brendan's idea of the profession: you've introduced the idea of public regard.

Doug: Exactly.

Chairman: How does the medical profession win that respect?

Tony: One of the reasons the medical profession is held in so much public regard is that they are a group of people who are reasonably well educated, and who have a lot of contact with people in the community. I think it's this close contact with people who they are trying to help which is at the root of the public's regard for the profession.

Chairman: Tony's point has been made by writers commenting on the high regard in which doctors were held in the latter part of the nineteenth century. When science became a force for social good, doctors were seen to be practical scientists who had direct contact with human beings, and whose activities could be appreciated by the man in the street.

Rod: As soon as something is labelled 'a profession' that tends to produce some regard. It produces a feeling that one should look up to the members of the profession. It implies something special.

Dave: Another point is that the basic activity of most professions tends to be direct involvement with people. That would be true of the medical profession, the legal profession, the teaching profession, and the church.

Chairman: Having acknowledged that, I could reply that a bus driver, a garbage man, and a football coach all have contact with people as an integral part of their vocational activity. Is it just contact with people that is basic to the concept of a profession?

Rod: I suppose we don't regard physiotherapy as a profession, and yet physiotherapists have closer contact with people and patients than doctors.

Nicholas: Part of the respect the public has for the medical profession comes from its mysticism. Although there is a contact between the profession and the public, it's a very unequal contact. The professional person has a special skill which the recipient doesn't have.

Chairman: You've made an interesting comment, Nick: you used the words 'mysticism' and 'special skill'. Did you mean both, or is there a difference?

Tony: It's skill from our point of view, but it's frequently mystic from the patient's point of view.

Chairman: That's a good answer. Is the concept of 'special skill' essential to the definition of the profession?

David: I think we're dealing with a very foggy area. Someone who is a plumber might regard themselves as a member of a profession while an outsider might regard them as a tradesman. Profession is a term I'd rather avoid, especially when talking about the medical profession.

Rod: Why?

David: Because I don't like to think that when I say, 'I'm a professional person and you're a tradesman', I imply 'therefore I'm better than you'. I don't like that.

Dave: But that's how it's developed.

David: It also implies certain responsibilities, particularly responsibilities to the other members of your profession.

Chairman: Well, David has put forward one response to the question, 'What does the concept of the profession imply?' What do others think?

Liz: The concept of the profession implies a responsibility to the community as well.

Doug: One special aspect of belonging to the medical profession is that people divulge their innermost secrets to you, and so they expect their doctor to be something special.

David: I still don't think you have to be called by a special name in order to be special. Many people would regard accountants, teachers, and architects as professionals and yet people don't necessarily go around divulging their innermost secrets to them. So that can't be a necessary part of the definition of a professional.

Chairman: David, I don't think that's quite the point. As a professional, certain things fall under your contract. For a doctor, one of those things is trust in relation to the secrets of your patients; particularly what the Hippocratic Oath called, 'not noising abroad whatsoever one hears or sees in relation to the private lives of one's patients'. If that is part of your professional covenant then to be a professional one must adhere to it. Now it may be that accountants, footballers, and actors have their own special requirements of behaviour. No one would suggest they should be the same as for doctors. No one would suggest that there should be cross reciprocation between the different professions on those specific requirements.

David: The point that I was trying to make was that just because you are called a member of a profession and certain things are required of your behaviour, I don't see how that makes a doctor a professional, and a plumber a tradesman. That's why I don't like the term 'professional'.

Tony: Some people think that 'profession' implies a conspiracy of silence, particularly in relation to the medical profession. A lot of people go to doctors not expecting to be told much. I believe some patients feel that doctors discuss their cases between themselves and then just return with the answer. Often there's very little dialogue between the patient and doctor.

Chairman: Bernard Shaw made a claim that 'all professions are conspiracies against the laity'. Do you think that's true?

Brendan: In one sense that is true, but it also works the other way. By being a member of a profession, a member has a moral obligation to keep up the standard of their performance. Now, no one is going to blame a plumber if he tells other people about the inner secrets of your plumbing; but I think the legal profession, accountants, and doctors all have additional obligations to their clients. This is an obligation in a moral sense, and not just in providing a service for a fee. There are other more personal aspects.

David: I disagree with that, because a plumber can see the innermost aspects of your home and you don't want him to go around telling Mrs Smith next door what was the state of hygiene in your house–how much butter was spilt on the carpet, or how many oranges were found blocking the toilet.

Brendan: But no one is going to think a plumber is terrible if he did.

David: I wouldn't be impressed. I feel it doesn't matter who we call a professional, after all, a plumber who has served an apprenticeship and has special skills can also be called a professional.

Chairman: Inherent in your contract as a doctor is the rule that you don't divulge the secrets of your patients to other people. Inherent in your professionalism as a plumber would be not to use a material which is unsafe–a particular pipe, or a certain cement–for example. The fact that a doctor can make his own plumbing modifications to his roof so that he can develop his own X-rays is not quite the important issue in relation to his professionalism, nor is the fact that a plumber has access to some of your secrets.

I take your point, David, but what I'd like us to concentrate on now is this: given that we use the term 'profession' in relation to medical doctors and nurses, what are the specific obligations for members of our profession? Just a few moments ago someone said that belonging to a profession implied a special skill or talent which no one else had, and that it required a high degree of training. What are some of the other good and bad points involved in the concepts of our profession?

Nicholas: I think one drawback of being a member of a profession is that it tends to make the individuals in that profession similar parts of a 'one'. The danger is that the 'one' fails to recognize that in a profession there will always be people with different abilities and different talents. If you label someone a member of a profession then you tend to attach certain characteristics to them which they might not have as individuals. Another point is that someone could hide their incompetence under the blanket of professionalism.

Chairman: Nicholas you said two things there: first, a doctor frequently has to submerge his individual personality and take on the professional personality–we discussed that in Session 3; and second, that certain less-talented, inadequate, ineffective, or inefficient members of the profession may hide under the corporate reputation of the profession.

Brendan: It works the other way too, in that an incompetent member can be excluded from a profession which controls its own standards of entrance. It's almost certain that if, as a result of your behaviour, the profession won't accept you, then society won't accept you as a doctor either. This will help to guard against the incompetence of certain members. I suppose it could also work the other way in that certain eccentric members are unjustifiably excluded.

Liz: Going on from Brendan's point, if there is an article in the paper about one incompetent doctor then there could be unjustified blanket criticism of the profession because of that one member's behaviour.

Chairman: Brendan touched on something new in his last comment: that the profession is responsible for its own standards, and is self-monitoring in relation to the behaviour and activities of its members. That doesn't necessarily apply to some of the other vocations which David mentioned in his opening comments. The medical profession will pass and fail its own members in examinations, and does have the power to withdraw registration from certain doctors whom it regards as unsatisfactory.

Tony: As it stands at the moment, professional self-monitoring only occurs in the early stages of a doctor's career. Once graduated, doctors don't have to sit exams to have their competence judged. That could allow all sorts of defects to creep in.

Brendan: And yet if a doctor doesn't perform well he can be called up before the Registration Board.

Tony: But it has to be a pretty gross misdemeanour before that happens.

Chairman: Does the group feel that the monitoring of doctors who are beyond university graduation is inadequate?

Dave: Yes.

Gillian: Yes.

Male Student: Yes.

Dave: In a way, the profession depends on a personal self-monitoring system. There is a very great obligation of conscience on a doctor to stay informed and competent. People in a particular profession like the medical profession are looked up to, and that respect should stimulate an obligation to maintain standards.

Chairman: What Matthew Arnold called '*noblesse oblige*' when referring to the aristocracy of England.

Gillian: Yes, it means to behave in a way that is noble in order to be treated in a noble fashion.

Chairman: What then are the specific responsibilities which would guarantee professional respect?

Hilary: It's as we've been saying. It's to behave in a way which will not detract from the standards society expects of the profession. The fact that you are held in respect by other members of the profession is important.

Chairman: There have been some moves to make a peer review compulsory. That is, doctors who have graduated must continue to formally show that they are maintaining an adequate standard of medical knowledge. Do you think this will come? And do you think the move will come from within the profession or without?

David: I don't think it will come from outside the profession because the profession just wouldn't accept it. And I think it's unlikely to come from within the profession for a very long time, so I can't see it happening in the near future.

Hilary: I think refresher courses would be a better idea than structured exams.

[*General agreement.*]

Jane: One of the disadvantages of being in a profession, is that one has to guard against becoming too far separated from the rest of the community.

Chairman: Do you think this is happening?

Jane: Yes I do.

Chairman: In which ways are we separate from society as a whole?

Rod: We don't get as many holidays!

Jane: The whole of health care revolves around the medical profession. I don't think this is such a good thing because there are many people outside the profession who have something to contribute to the problem of health care. I think that specialized care must come from the medical profession, but that other areas need not. Too much centralization of health care within the medical profession is bad.

Chairman: Are there any qualities intrinsic to our profession which separate us from normal members of society?

Nicholas: As doctors we have to face up to many ugly aspects of life such as sickness and death. Most people in the medical profession accept death as an everyday event, and yet for the average member of society the death of a relative only happens two or three times in their lifetime.

Chairman: So there are stresses on us, stresses that are not shared by individuals at large, but which we might share with certain other professions.

Rod: Sickness is something which people outside the profession tend to run away from. I think one of the reasons we're looked up to by members of society is that we put up with their troubles, and we have to deal with them because we can't run away from them. It's our job.

Jane: Another responsibility of being a member of the medical profession is that people expect the doctor to be able to understand and cure what's going wrong with them.

Rod: For a medical student that's one of the really demoralizing things about doing medicine, the fact that you find out very quickly that there are so many diseases a doctor can't do anything about; so many conditions for which we just treat the symptoms with pain-killers or something like that.

Chairman: That is an important point. I think many members of society still think in terms of a magic cure for their condition. But if one adds up the number of conditions in practice where a specific cause is known, and therefore specific treatment is possible, they number only four or five: the infectious diseases, the specific nutritional deficiencies, the endocrine diseases, some surgical cases like trauma, and perhaps, in future, the inborn errors of metabolism.

Now let us change direction. When did the modern medical profession start? I mean, to which time can we trace the present governing statutes of our profession?

Gillian: Was it the sixteenth century?

Chairman: Yes, I think one could say when Dr Thomas Linacre came back from the Italian medical schools in the latter part of the fifteenth century and became physician to Henry VIII, he used his influence to convince King Henry that there was a need for improvement and uniformity of standards in the medical guild. Young King Henry agreed, and the original statutes of the College of Physicians were set up in the early 1500s. In many ways one could regard Henry VIII as the father of the modern medical profession.

Let us consider an extract from the early parliamentary Act which led to the foundation of the original College of Physicians six years later. The Act of 1511 contains the reasons why the original college was set up, and was the first parliamentary enactment about medical affairs.

> The science and cunning of physick and surgery (to the perfect knowledge whereof be requisite both great learning and ripe experience) is daily within the realm exercised by a great multitude of ignorant persons of whom the greater part have no manner of insight in the same, nor any other kind of learning . . . in the which they partly use sorcery and witchcraft, partly apply such medicines unto the disease as be very noxious . . . [to] the grievous hurt, damage, and destruction of many of the King's liege people.[1]

Gillian: What this passage is saying is that in 1511 the opportunity to practise medicine was available to everyone, but that it should have been limited because a lot of harm was being done to the public. It's also saying the practice of medicine requires great learning.

Chairman: So in this early statute we have the ideas behind why this profession came into existence. First, to protect patients against individuals who were not capable of looking after them; and second, the recognition that to practise medicine requires special knowledge and training. However, thirty-two years later in 1543, another Act was passed. I believe this extract from the Act contains the germs of two problems which have plagued the medical profession for the following four centuries.

> Since the making of the original Act, the company and fellowship of the surgeons of London, mindful only of their own lucres, and nothing of the profit of the diseases or patient, have sued, troubled, and vexed various divers honest persons, as well as men and women, whom God hath endued with the knowledge of the nature, kind and operation of certain herbs, roots and waters . . . and yet the said (honest) persons have not taken anything for their labours or cunning, but have ministered the same to poor people only for neighbourhood and God's sake and pity and charity.[2]

Stuart: This Act admits that many people who were doing good have been excluded from the practice of medicine, and sets out to correct that injustice. Those who were excluded under the general headings of 'sorcery and witchcraft' are now admitted as 'various divers honest persons who have a knowledge of herbs'. It's also saying that many of the people who were banned were behaving more altruistically than the medical profession itself.

Gillian: It seems the people who have been chosen as professional members have been taking advantage of their status.

David: It's interesting that this Act refers to the Company and Fellowship of Surgeons of London, and not the members of the original College of Physicians. One of the points that the second passage makes is that it asks whether or not the medical profession is basically altruistic or basically a business like anything else.

Tony: It's also making another point: how much are we (the medical profession) justified in restricting the activities of other people whose talents may overlap with ours? In the case of the medical profession in the sixteenth century it was the herbalists, these days one could say it is the chiropractors or the acupuncturists.

Chairman: Tony's point has identified one of the two major criticisms contained in this passage: our intolerance of people who are outside our profession but whose area of interest overlaps. Is there a second point which has some modern relevance?

Tony: Yes, surgeons are mindful only of their own financial interests.

Brendan: This brings in another aspect of professionalism. One tends to think of a doctor as someone who is not just doing a job working for money. But it's disheartening that there are a lot of doctors who *do* espouse this as their aim. I think that inherent in the idea of being a member of the medical profession is the belief that you're doing a worthwhile job, and that earning your living is not the prime consideration. Obviously everyone has to earn their living, but the primary motivation for doctors should not be one of financial reward. It would be appalling if doctors, like footballers, switched jobs just because of the possibility of increased financial reward. A professional person in medicine should be dedicated in both the scientific and moral sense. According to that view I suppose there are a lot of unprofessional people in medicine, and in many other professions. I know a number of student colleagues who have openly admitted that they're only doing medicine in order to make money. I think that's very sad.

David: I don't think there's anybody in their right mind who would do medicine just to make money, because there are many easier methods of becoming rich than being a doctor. After all, you spend six years doing a course for which you are paid nothing, when you could be exploring other methods of making money. Medicine is not the way to get rich.

Jane: I disagree. It's relative; after all, doctors make a lot more money than labourers, tradesmen, and members of other professions. Doctors seem to have plenty of money to live on.

Brendan: Medicine does imply that once you've graduated, provided you can stick the course out, you've always got a job guaranteed. One of the students the other day was criticizing some labourers for leaning on shovels, and I asked them, 'If you were offered $1000 a week to work as a wharfie would you go and do it?' and a lot of them said, 'Yes.' I find that very sad in a sense, because if somebody's not dedicated to their profession and to their studies, then I don't think they're in the right place, and they can't be good doctors.

Chairman: I think Brendan made a good point when he said none of us are going to be economically threatened during our lives. The qualification of medical doctor does guarantee us considerable financial security, and also vocational security. None of us will ever be made redundant, and barring some major misdemeanour we're never going to be sacked. Now that's a very privileged position for an individual to be in these days with the current economic climate.

Hilary: If anyone did do medicine for purely financial security reasons, I think they would find the drain of the demands of being a doctor so great they'd probably give it up.

Chairman: Either that, or they might start to cut corners and become remote; their performance could become bad.

Brendan: Or they might join a group practice and work from nine to five.

David [*indignantly*]: Well what's wrong with that?

Brendan: Nothing.
David: Well you've just been pouring absolute venom . . .
Brendan: I'm pouring venom on anybody who does a professional course for purely financial reasons.
Chairman: David, do you think such an approach is compatible with professionalism?
David: No, but I don't think anybody does any job purely for money . . .

[*General disagreement.*]

Male student: It's a matter of degree.
Brendan: I don't want to repeat myself, but anyone who does medicine should be doing it for better reasons than financial gain.
Stuart: It's very difficult to be sure of your motivations when you're eighteen years of age, they may change during the course or afterwards.
Brendan: That's all very well. But what about the nine students who missed out on selection for the one who got in? Amongst the ones who were rejected there may have been quite a number who wanted to be doctors for better motives and who would have been better doctors.
Chairman: Stuart, just don't cast your eyes to the ceiling in disgust, say something.
David: If you're competent, what the hell does it matter what your motivation is?
Brendan [*raising his voice*]*:* But it does, it does, it reflects on your attitudes.
Hilary: You can't be competent without motivation.
Tony: Competence extends to more things than just a knowledge of a few simple routines. The practice of medicine is more than just what drug to give for 'this' and what symptoms are associated with 'that'. It's much more than that.
Jane: I don't see how anyone who has special skills should expect excessive financial returns for doing something to help other people–people who don't have the skills. It seems dreadful that you should be remunerated to an excessive degree because of the suffering of others.
Rod: All jobs are remunerated.
Jane: But not to the same extent as doctors . . .
Rod: The guy who presses the button in a factory, he's doing a job for other people too, isn't he?
Jane [*persisting*]*:* I don't see how you can morally justify being rewarded excessively for having a skill which society has paid for you to have.
Chairman: What is the justification for the members of the medical

profession being in an economically privileged position? Jane is saying there is none. Who can answer that?

Rod: I don't know if they *are* in an economically privileged position. You take a first-year intern at this hospital; even if he's earning $20 000 a year or something like that, if you work it out on an hourly rate he's earning about $2.30 an hour. Now you show me . . .

Chairman: With respect Rod, I think you're begging the point. If one looks at the salaries which doctors earn in relation to other members of society, or the houses they live in, or the cars they drive, or the schools they send their children to, or the number of overseas trips they take, then you'll see that doctors *are* in a relatively privileged financial position. Now the question for us is, 'Is that justified?'

Rod: Well I think they deserve it because they work harder than everyone else. They certainly work harder than forty hours a week.

Brendan: I can point to plenty of Italian people who work in factories for more than forty hours a week and they certainly don't get the returns that doctors do. I can point to Australians who drive taxis till 1.00 a.m. every day, and they certainly don't get the rate that doctors do.

Rod: I didn't say that I don't believe that doctors are in an economically privileged position, I'm just saying that maybe it's justified.

David: Nobody would dispute the fact that doctors are economically privileged. As to whether or not they should be or not, that's a different question.

Chairman: Well, Jane says they shouldn't be.

David: Then you have to consider your whole philosophy of whether or not you feel that everybody in society is entitled to high economic privileges, or whether you think that people should be paid for the amount of work they do, or for the amount of training they've put in. Obviously the community at the moment agrees that if you do put in a lot of training, and work hard, you will finish up with a lot of money. Now whether or not you *should* is a basic philosophical question.

Chairman: Where do you stand on it?

David: I think that if you work hard for the money then you probably deserve it. Although I think there's a cut-off above which no one should be entitled to it. For example, I don't believe in money making money.

Liz: I support what David has said. I've spoken to a lot of people who say that doctors deserve the money they get because they've done a six-year course, they do work hard and they do get up at night. That's perhaps not my own personal view, but that's what is said.

Chairman: What is your view?

Liz: Well that's a very hard question to answer.

Hilary: In any job situation in the community there should be incentives to work hard and to work well. That can apply to medicine, and . . .

Jane: Why does the incentive need to be a financial one?

Hilary: I'm not saying it has to be.

Tony: There are better rewards than the financial ones for a doctor.

Nicholas: I think it's pretty terrible if you're so undedicated that you need money to stimulate you to work.

Chairman: What is evil about money?

Gillian: Yes, we're all implying that earning money is something bad.

Jane: It's not evil in itself. But where you have some individuals in society who have so much money that they don't know what to do with it, the inequality can be evil.

Tony: It would be very interesting to do a cost effectiveness study on the medical profession to see what it earns, how much money it consumes, and what good it produces. It would be interesting to know where doctors put their money. I think there are better rewards for dedication and hard work than money, and I think the medical profession has concentrated too much on money and financial reward for what they do. It would be better if they took a less acquisitive point of view on economic matters.

Stuart: You have to look at the whole employment structure in our society to gain some indication of where doctors fit. I don't support the view that money should be the only reward that doctors seek; but we *are* talking about money. Now if you look at the top jobs, you've got things like aircraft pilots, engineers, architects, most of the professions.

Chairman [*interrupting*]*:* And doctors at the top. There have been published figures which suggest that, on average earning, the members of the medical profession come out on top of the professions in terms of economic reward.

Stuart: Well it makes no difference to my argument because the criteria which set that scale could be things like the amount of stress which an individual is under. I mean the obvious case is an airline pilot or someone like that. Someone like pilots would get more money because they have a considerable amount of responsibility, their vocational life ends at forty, and they have to go through as much training as we do. So it's important they are well paid while they're working.

Chairman: What would you say to the proposition that, unlike the airline pilot, the doctor has got a captive clientele? If you're ill you have to go and see a doctor, but if you want to travel, you don't have to go by an aeroplane?

[*Wild comment and disagreement*] That's irrelevant!

Dave: Could I put in a couple of comments? Last weekend I picked up a couple of hitch-hikers who were on their way to the beach. One of them was a brickie, the other one was an apprentice tradesman. When I told them I was at the university doing medicine they said, 'Oh, you'll be a doctor one day, you'll earn plenty of money.' They both agreed that because of the amount of training we have to do and the amount of responsibility we have when we graduate, the money doctors get was entirely justified.

Chairman: What do you feel about that?

Dave: I think I agree with it.

Nicholas: Can I put forward an alternative. What we've just been doing is discussing basic Western society. There's a lot more to the world than that. In our society we seem to think that money is the centre of rewards. But what about a lot of countries where doctors have a reasonable professional status and aren't necessarily rewarded highly in terms of money. For instance, in the U.S.S.R. doctors don't receive very much money at all, and are on the same level of salaries as teachers, but I don't think their professionalism or their professional status suffers because they aren't getting a lot of money. Just before [*to the chairman*] you asked was there anything evil about money. I think it is evil because it tends to produce the sort of metamorphosis described in one of the passages from Session 3. When somebody starts going all out for money, they become unprofessional through the desire for riches. Could anyone answer, 'Why is money so essential as an incentive?'

Doug: I recently saw an article about corruption in medicine in the U.S.S.R. It described how there were many people paying lots of money to get their children into medicine.

Chairman: You seemed to have said two things Doug. First, that Nicholas's view of Russian medicine may be rather starry-eyed, but the more important and fundamental point is that you're saying this is an example of the 'evils' of money, which was precisely the point that Nicholas was making. So you're agreeing with him?

[*General laughter.*]

Doug [*laughing*]*:* Yes, I suppose I am.

Rod: You only have to go back to the first page of the Bible to sort this out. The reason we're down here on earth and not up there in heaven is because Adam took the bite out of the apple. Man is naturally a selfish, greedy person.

Chairman: Yeah Rod, but not all of us are as hung up on that Christian belief. [*Laughter.*] I feel that the opinion that man is basically evil is the greatest 'con' that has ever been put on to mankind, and is one of the greatest forces for evil. The Greeks believed that a man with self-respect for his own achivement, and whose ego meant self-esteem and self-fulfilment, had pride and force and power. Perhaps the ideal of a man striving to contribute the maximum he is capable of is the one we should look to, and not the Christian idea where every time a man is humble, or self-negating, or self-effacing, he's considered to be expressing great virtue.

Rod: Well, I wasn't saying that.

Chairman: But it's implicit in the point you put that man is basically born evil.

Rod: All *I'm* saying is that man *is* basically evil.

Chairman: Well *I'm* saying he *isn't*. I'm saying more than that. I'm saying that probably the Christian outlook has brainwashed you but hasn't brainwashed me.

[*Cheering and applause.*]

Gillian: Pick yourself up, Rod.

Rod: Geez!

Brendan: In part I agree; the excuse of man's basically evil nature has been one of the great justifications for greediness.

Rod: Well I don't know if 'evil' is the right word, but I believe that man is basically selfish. Even the most selfless person is getting satisfaction out of what he's doing, so basically he's selfish. Even when he's helping others he's getting an ego kick for himself so he's really doing it for himself.

Chairman: Rod, you have put forward an argument which has been put forward by philosophers. This 'self-love' 'social-love' argument was debated at length in the early part of the eighteenth century. And the point which you made was argued by a very clever fellow called Bernard de Mandeville in this book *The Fable of the Bees*. But it's a circular argument: if you say that every time a man does something which is truly benevolent he really is selfish because he's taking quiet satisfaction in the fact that he's done something benevolent, then that point can't be argued against.

Gillian: I think it's easier to explain . . . I mean it's easy for *me* to explain to myself why people do things on the basis of selfishness than any other motive.

Rod: Another point I'd like to make is if a doctor in practice believes that money isn't the prime reward for his services, then there's nothing to stop him not taking it.

Chairman: Can I introduce a little bit of history here by reading a letter which was published this week in the *Medical Journal of Australia*; the heading is 'Greedy Doctors, Unjustified Claim'.

Sir:
Accusations of financial greed, such as we have heard recently, tend to turn the stomach of doctors, or raise their gall, or even make them a little testy. Surgeons tend to become defensive and even a little irritated at these unjustified and unwarranted criticisms. So the purpose of this letter is certainly not to rap the ever-so-talented knuckles of our surgeons.

I believe there is such a thing as a professional personality, which has all of the complexities and intrigues of an individual one. Many perceptive writers and wits have noticed the blemishes in our professional personality: our hostility towards outsiders; our professional conservatism; and our mistrust of the non-scientific. They have even noticed our professional mammonism.

I do not think our profession realizes just how ingrained and recurrent has been the charge of greed against doctors in virtually every century. The grasping affinities of surgeons 'mindful of their own lucres, and nothing the profit of the patient or disease' were noted in the earliest Acts of Henry VIII, which set up the original Royal College of Physicians in the early part of the sixteenth century; and the charge has been repeated in every following century by a whole library of authors. Francis Bacon described that 'the characteristic beneficience of the profession is inconsistent with a sordid view and avaricious rapacity'. And Montaigne's view that doctors 'consider their own reputation and consequently their profit rather than their patients' interest' is the one which has clung to the profession from Aristophanes to A. J. Cronin. In medieval England, the system of payment was determined by the patient's satisfaction with his cure, but John of Salisbury suggested that 'where poverty is, labour is not worthwhile for the doctor', and that 'doctors should take their fee while the patient is sick', thereby earning the rebuke:

> But, when that cure complete, he seeks his fee,
> The Devil looks less terrible than he.

Sancho Panza observed that 'a doctor gives advice by the pulse of your pocket'. And Dr Tobias Smollett's character, Dr Fathom, took the title of Doctor 'to insinuate himself into the pockets of his patients'. Like Smollett, Samuel Garth was a doctor, and in his celebrated poem, *The Dispensary*, he struck out at the mean behaviour of doctors who had refused to treat the poor of London without charge:

> Though doctors differ,
> In this one point they never disagree,
> They are all unanimous about the fee. . . .
> Think on the meed that tickles sweet your hand,
> The glittering meed, no doctor can withstand . . .
> How fighting Physic hangs her pensive head,
> And what was once a Science, now is a trade.

> If there is a current public sentiment which regards doctors somewhat ambiguously in relation to their preoccupation with fees (and I believe there is), then those who regard such charges as unfair need to recall the traditional public attitude, and need to acknowledge that traditional social attitudes, which have evolved out of the past always reflect some truth.[3]

Brendan: That sounds like it's been written by a friend of ours.

Stuart: It certainly sounds familiar.

Gillian: There couldn't be too many who could have written that!

Chairman: Yes, of course I wrote it, and I present it now to put forward another point. Irrespective of what *we* believe on the justice of doctors' claims for this fee or that fee, there is a background of public hostility against the medical profession in relation to its preoccupation with money. Irrespective of how misinformed or how true it is, this public sentiment is a factor to be considered in any negotiations by doctors on money. Whenever doctors embark on discussions with governments on the question of payments those discussions take place against a background of hypersensitivity on this issue.

Nicholas: I think your point of view is essentially correct. Although people tend to regard their own doctor in a certain way, when the profession is taken as a whole the public are far less happy. The public thinks that the medical profession is a money-grabbing lot of bastards. The public sees the medical profession driving around in Rolls Royces and Mercedes, they see the big flash offices, and there may be some jealousy of this status.

Stuart [*to the chairman*]*:* Are you suggesting the medical profession should use its wit in such negotiations?

Chairman: I think we've got to approach this area delicately. Allergic reactions only need a tiny stimulus to set them off.

Rod: Another interesting point came out of that letter. When people are sick they don't mind paying the doctor however much they ask because they think they're going to get something out of it; but once they're well again they forget what's been done for them.

David: Perhaps we should work on the imperial Chinese system where the patient only paid the doctor while he was well, and stopped paying him when he got ill.

[*Laughter.*]

Brendan: I don't think many people are upset by the high wages of doctors because many others in society are on high wages. People get very sensitive when doctors make special excuses for why they deserve to be paid more, such as they've studied for a long time, or they have to get up at night, and that sort of thing. That seems to me to reduce the profession to the level of a trade. Now I enjoy studying and I think my studentship is going to be the easiest time in my life. People who crap on about how much sacrifice they made during their student years make me sick.

Tony: I agree, I think my university days are so valuable and they are days which I enjoy.

Hilary: It would be nice if there was more financial ease about those days though. I wouldn't mind being paid a bit more now and a bit less later on so that I don't have to worry about the rent.

Stuart: I don't share Brendan and Tony's attraction to the joys of university life. And I agree with Hilary that I would like to feel a little more financially secure during the six years of the medical course. I basically just don't have an affinity for studying.

Gillian: I'd like to ask a question. Do you think it's possible that someone could be a better doctor because they are paid more?

Chairman: What's your answer to your own question?

Gillian: Maybe the fact that a doctor is paid a lot of money makes him a better doctor because it makes him more secure. I think perhaps it might; but I don't think it justifies the incredibly high salaries which some doctors earn.

Chairman: Am I understanding you correctly Gillian—are you saying that an adequate amount of financial security for a doctor would help to eliminate greed and free his life from purely financial pursuits?

Gillian: Yes I am. And so that would make him a better doctor.

Nicholas: That all sounds cosy. But that's not the real-life situation. A certain level of financial remuneration is reasonable, I don't think anybody would argue against that. The centre of the discussion is whether or not we need the constant incentive of more and more money. If I could just go on with this discussion of money in medicine, can anyone justify better health care for better money?

David: What do you mean? Are you asking, 'Should a patient be able to get better health care just because he's rich?'

Nicholas: Yes, I am.

David: As a basis for medical practice I think that it's totally unacceptable. There should be equal availability of health care irrespective of financial status.

Rod: I agree that for more money to equal better health care sounds really bad. But there are situations where company directors get sent overseas to America by their firms for better treatment. Now, we can't send all of the patients we'd like to over to a specialist centre for specialist treatment because there just isn't the money available. So sometimes the situation does arise where someone who has the money to pay for treatment can get it. In that way you can have a situation where more money does equal better treatment.

Nicholas: I don't see how that justifies it.

David: That boils down to 'Should anyone have that much money?'

Nicholas: It's one thing to have a rare example, but that's not the rule.

Tony: Can I recount an example of something that happened recently? A surgeon in Casualty walked up to a patient who had acute abdominal pain and said to him as he was writhing around, 'Now do you want to be a private patient or a public patient? The nursing care's the same, but if you're a private patient I'll take an extra special interest in you'. What he was implying was, 'If you're a private patient I'd *really* look after you!" Now I thought that was disgusting.

Rod: I think that's terrible.

Doug: When a doctor attacks somebody when they're sick and vulnerable they'd grasp for any treatment they think is better. That really is ugly exploitation.

Chairman: There *is* vulnerability in illness, and perhaps some of the health companies who are advertising health coverage are preying on those fears. You know the sort of thing: 'Are you *sure* your family has got adequate health cover?'

Brendan: Could I make one more point, I think the taxpayer spends about $70 000 in training each of us. Most of us have a good time, I think it's fair to say; [*looking across at Stuart*] it's unfortunate if you don't. We should go out into the community not thinking that the community owes us something but that we owe the community something back.

Chairman: This point was made in one of Brecht's plays, I think it was *Mother Courage*, in which a doctor was told by the peasants, 'We educated you, now you care for us, we are responsible for your position, you are obliged to us.'

Brendan: The way I feel, it's public money that put us through university.

Rod: But most of that public money has come from the taxes on doctors who are earning all that money.

[*General moan.*]

Chairman: Now, does anyone want to take up the other criticism which was implied in those early sixteenth-century statutes, that is, that the profession is intolerant of 'outsiders'?

David: There's a good and a bad side to that. The bad side is that the profession says let's have the field to ourselves and get rid of any competitors because they take work away from us. The good side involves a concern for patients in that you won't have people who are ignorant of underlying medical conditions looking after you. I mean a chiropractor could manipulate a spine which is really the seat of a secondary tumour.

Chairman: I agree with that point; if there's something wrong with one's car one doesn't leave it to the man who serves petrol, one takes it to the mechanic. Similarly, if one has a headache it might be something which a chiropractor could do something for, but it could also be the start of a brain tumour, malignant hypertension, or even an aneurysm. David's point is fundamentally true and is related to that aspect of professionalism which we considered earlier under technical or special expertise.

Tony: On the other hand we looked at examples last week of people who were sent to doctors with psychological problems and the doctor's first response was to do a physical examination and to look at things only in a medical context. That's a very narrow approach.

Nicholas: Another bad aspect is the abuse of the closed shop. There have been cases where overseas graduates have been excluded from practice here because they don't have local degrees.

Chairman: Hang on a moment Nicholas, I think that's irrelevant to the point we're discussing. I thought you were going to talk about the concept of a closed shop. What you've given us is an example of the profession monitoring its own standards. I mean one could commend the profession for making sure that all its members were up to scratch.

Nicholas: I don't necessarily agree. After all a doctor who is not part of the local scene can be treated very much as an outsider.

Gillian: But if he's going to be capable of practising in the local scene he's got to come up to the local standards.

Jane: I don't think the medical profession makes a big enough effort in trying to work together with other disciplines which are related to medicine.

Chairman: Someone once said that the medical profession's hostility towards an outside group is directly proportional to their own lack of performance in the area which the outside group is involved with.

David: That's true to some extent, I suppose the reason that chiropractors do so well is that doctors are not very good at treating back injuries.

Chairman: Let's change our approach now and consider a passage from George Eliot's fine novel, *Middlemarch*. It discusses the relationship between patients, and doctors within the profession.

> 'Lydgate has lots of ideas quite new about ventilation and diet and that sort of thing.' . . .
>
> 'Hang it, do you think that is quite sound?—upsetting the old treatment, which has made Englishmen what they are?' said Mr Standish.
>
> 'Medical knowledge is at a low ebb among us,' said Mr Bulstrode,

> who spoke in a subdued tone, and had a rather sickly air. 'I, for my part, hail the event of Dr Lydgate.' . . .
>
> 'That's all very fine,' replied Mr Standish, who was not fond of Mr Bulstrode; 'if you like him to try experiments on your hospital patients, and kill a few people for charity, I have no objection. But I am not going to have money out of my purse to have experiments tried on me. I like treatment that has been tested a little.
>
> 'Well you know Standish, every dose you take is an experiment,' said Mr Brooke . . .[4]

David: This is the classic problem of the new idea being received with hostility and anger. This has happened all through medical and scientific history. When Galileo said that the earth went around the sun and not the opposite, he was threatened with the torture of an inquisition. He was forced to renounce because it upset the establishment ideas. This is the same thing–the people in this passage have their comfortable ideas and Doctor Lydgate is coming in with his new ideas about ventilation and diet and they find it threatening.

Chairman: Do you think the medical profession has a strong tradition of this sort of conservatism?

David: Yes.

Chairman: Well what are the good aspects of our professional conservatism?

David: Scientific conservatism will prevent tragedies like Thalidomide occurring again. It prevents drugs which may be dangerous from being used before they are fully tested. That could also be bad in that drugs like aspirin and penicillin wouldn't get on the market now if they had to be put through today's rigorous drug tests.

Chairman: What are some of the other expressions of conservatism in medicine?

David: Well there's the red-necked irrational conservatism. When Lister was advocating antisepsis, surgeons used to make jokes and say, 'Shut the door in case any of Lister's organisms get in'. When the profession rejects a doctor or a discovery without examining the objective evidence they can do medicine a great disservice.

Chairman: As with the response to Simpson, Pasteur, and Semmelweis.

What about political conservatism? Let me play the 'Devil's advocate'. What if I were to say that 85 per cent of doctors in Britain, Australia, Canada, and the U.S.A. are politically conservative, that is, they vote for conservative parties, and yet in each of these countries the public which they serve is about equally divided between left- and right-wing sympathies. What is the significance of that political disproportion between the medical profession and the public?

Jane: A potential problem could arise if doctors used their position to try and impose their own political view on their patients . . .

Rod: Oh come on! How many doctors have a sign, when you walk in, which says, 'Unless you vote conservative I won't treat you.'

Jane [*not flustered*]*:* Just a moment. I'll give you some examples. A patient who was a conscientious objector against the war in Vietnam went to a doctor with a genuine medical complaint and the doctor turned around and said he thought he was weak and cowardly and ought to go and fight in Vietnam.

Doug: That's just one case.

Chairman: Perhaps so; but recently I came upon a newspaper report from 1951 where there was actually a meeting of doctors in this city [Melbourne] to decide whether or not the medical profession ought to report to the government any patient who had extreme left-wing sympathies.

Dave: Really?

Stuart: That's unbelievable. Was it symptomatic of the era?

Chairman: It was symptomatic of the era, but that's just the point. We have no protection against such an era returning.

Rod: If I could just give an answer to Jane. I think that a lot of people from a lot of other professions would have said the same thing to conscientious objectors. I don't think you can say that doctors as a profession use their position to influence people's political ideas.

Jane: Well *you've* been saying that doctors have a *special* position in society whereby people respect them. I'm saying that they shouldn't use this position of respect to influence people whose opinions differ from themselves. Now, I've given you an example of where one of them did.

Rod: A plumber might to the same thing.

Jane: But you've just said that plumbers don't have the same public trust as doctors.

Dave: Looking at it from a broader moral position, this political issue is a bit of a worry. The sort of thing that Jane has just described just shouldn't happen.

Doug: A patient would be pretty gullible if he could be influenced by a doctor's political opinion.

Chairman: That's at an individual level. But all of us would concede that medicine and politics do overlap in certain areas. Surely in those areas this disproportion in the political opinions of doctors could be a factor in negotiations with government, especially in relation to public health projects.

Stuart: But even at an individual level, doctors *do* influence their patients. After all, doctors can influence their patients to give up smoking, or to alter their lifestyle, or their marital relationships. It would seem to me that political influence wouldn't be all that far removed from those things.

Jane: There have been recent reports in the paper of doctors refusing to treat patients who had only government health insurance, and who didn't have private health cover.

Nicholas: I was sitting in an Outpatients session last term with a doctor who was asked by the patient, 'Should I stay in the government health scheme or should I have private health insurance?' The doctor gave an answer which I believe was highly political. I think that situation is repeated time and time again all over the place. The doctor shouldn't be political in that situation, he can say, 'It's up to you to decide and here is my opinion.'

Chairman: Could I put a question to the group? I've only recently come back to Australia so I wasn't here during the height of the health scheme [Medibank] argument between the government and the profession. You were all here. On balance, do you think that the standing of the medical profession rose, stayed the same, or fell, as a result of that debate?

Brendan: The profession has come out of it with mud on its face. All of this propaganda and rubbish put out by the doctors on how Medibank was going to destroy health care was proven to be a whole lot of nonsense when the health scheme came in.

Tony: A couple of years ago, when I was interested in the Medibank issue, I went down to the Australian Medical Association office to get their literature on it. It was full of the most incredible distortions. It was full of propaganda and character assassinations. It was a disgrace.

Jane: I think the way the professions carried on could do nothing but make public regard for them go down.

Nicholas: A couple of weeks ago in this course we discussed trust. We discussed the error of the absolute lie and the error of omission which could take place between a doctor and a patient. I think the medical profession relies on honesty, that's one of the major qualities of professionalism. And yet over this health scheme issue we had the situation where doctors were very much lying to the public. I think that was proven because we had a year of efficient and good health care under Medibank. All of their predictions turned out to be untrue.

Rod: I also think the medical profession has lost a lot of face over the Medibank issue. But I disagree that Medibank made no difference to the practice of medicine. Because more patients went to see their doctors as a result of Medibank, many doctors were overworked and became taxed.

Chairman: If we had it over again and you were in charge of the profession's Medibank negotiations, what would you do differently to what was done last time?

Rod: I'm not sure, but I think what we've got now is worse than it has ever been; this mix-up of government health scheme and private health scheme is just a mess.

David: I agree, what we've finished up with now in this country is just the most ridiculous aggregation of bureaucratic nonsense that I've ever experienced. I think the medical profession made a complete fool of itself over this issue. All of the propaganda which was parcelled out, all the fears which were planted in the public mind, all of the leading advertisements which were placed in papers saying that this was going to distort and destroy the doctor-patient relationship with the poor mother and child being threatened with the dread hand of the socialist government, was absolute nonsense.

Hilary: This was the behaviour of the group of doctors who felt very threatened.

David: Yes, I agree, but they were a group of doctors who were threatened because they had vested interests in private health funds.

Stuart: I think this goes back to something we were saying earlier. I think the profession has lost face over Medibank, but it's a conservative profession and it dislikes change. Secondly, it was a change associated with money. As we've discussed before, it was bound to produce a reaction from the profession.

Chairman: That's an important point too, Stuart: one could argue that had the parliamentarians been a little better informed on the history and traditions of the medical profession, they would not have proceeded the way they did. Because both of these were sensitive areas to the medical profession, perhaps the negotiations could have been handled with greater delicacy on the part of the government.

Gillian: A lot of the public had made up their mind on what the doctors' reaction was going to be without giving them a chance to respond in a natural way. I don't think the public had an attitude of neutrality towards the profession to start with, it was one of aggression. Both sides were completely unreasonable about the whole situation.

Doug: There's no doubt our professionalism suffered over this Medibank issue. The medical profession was seen as a great big business interest.

Hilary: The whole exercise was a feat of poor organization from every direction. It seems to me that it would have been difficult to make it much better because of the basic hostilities and prejudices on both sides.

Chairman: Well, we're coming now to the last passage for today. It is one that attempts to capture the relationship between medicine and society. It's from Anton Chekhov's short story 'House with an Attic'. Two characters are involved in an argument: a young woman called Leda, and an unnamed artist.

> 'Last week Anna died in childbirth; if there had been a medical centre there she would be alive now. It seems to me that even landscape painters ought to have some convictions on this point.'
>
> 'I have most definite convictions on this point, I assure you,' I replied, while she concealed herself behind the newspaper, as though not wishing to listen to me. 'In my opinion, medical centres, schools, village libraries and dispensaries, under present conditions, merely serve the cause of enslavement. The people are entangled in a great chain, and you are not cutting through the chain but merely adding new links to it–there you have my conviction.'
>
> She raised her eyes, looked at me, and smiled sardonically, but I went on, trying to elucidate my main idea.
>
> 'What is important,' I said. 'is not that Anna died in childbirth, but that all these Annas, Mavras, and Pelageyas break their backs from morning till night, fall ill from work which is beyond their strength, are all their lives worrying over their sick and starving children, and all their lives afraid of death and disease, are all their lives looking for remedies for their illnesses, fade early, age early, and die in filth and stench. When they grow up, their children start the same thing all over again; and so centuries pass, and millions of people live worse than beasts, and all for a crust of bread–living in a state of continual fear. . . . Hunger, cold, animal fear, never-ending toil, have, like avalanches of snow, barred their way to spiritual activities, to the very thing that distinguishes man from the dumb beast and makes life worth living. You go their aid with hospitals and schools, but you don't free them from their fetters by that. On the contrary, you enslave them still more, for by introducing new standards into their life, you increase the number of their needs, . . .
>
> 'I'm not going to argue with you,' said Leda, putting down the paper. 'I've heard all this before, I will say only one thing: you can't just sit about and do nothing. It's true we are not saving humanity, and perhaps we make a great many mistakes; but we do all we can, and–we're right. The highest and most sacred task of civilized man is to serve his neighbours, and we try to serve them as best we can. You don't like it, but then one can't please everybody. . . . People usually say such charming things when they wish to justify their indifferences,' said Leda. 'To deny the usefulness of hospitals and schools is easier than to cure or to teach.'[5]

David: The artist seems to be putting forward a point of view similar to Ivan Illich; this could be a passage out of *Medical Nemesis*.

Rod: These days doctors are thinking more along the lines of prevention rather than cure.

[*Disagreement.*]

Nicholas: That's only a small point. What I think the writer is saying here is much more profound. The point of the artist's argument is that, at the moment, medicine is picking up what society has dropped, or what society has produced. So many sicknesses are just casualties of society. What the artist is recommending is that we should aim to change the whole of society and not just rely on the medical profession to patch things up. I think both people in this passage have similar goals, but they represent the conflict of the practitioner and the conceptual thinker. It's the conflict between the person at ground level who is trying to do practical things and the abstract thinker who's trying to generalize. I think both points are equally valid. One is doing something practical about an evil, i.e. palliation, and the other is trying to change the source of the evil.

Brendan: The artist seems to be putting forward the view of the armchair revolutionary and he's answered in the second-last sentence: ' "People usually say such charming things when they wish to justify their indifferences" '.

Chairman: In terms of modern relevance, which would you say were the areas where the medical profession is propping up the ills of society?

Rod: Something like cigarette smoking and lung cancer. There are two ways of curing lung cancer, simplistic ways like trying to chop it out, and the other way is to try to stop people smoking.

Tony: We also prop up the industrial society. Medicine as it is practised today is another device by which people are deluded into a belief that people care for them; just like they believe that the industrial society is doing better for them than would an agrarian way of life.

Gillian: This is such a well-balanced passage that it's difficult to argue with it.

Chairman: That's true, Chekhov did have an ability to put two sides of an argument through the characters. But still, we can ask the question, 'Which side is more relevant for us today?'

Gillian: I think the girl with her practical approach would be more relevant today.

David: Leda is talking about 'what I can do myself now', and the artist is saying what we must do to change society. In a sense they're talking on different levels.

Tony: A concern about what we can do now to prop up society is obscuring the big question. It's saying that we'll forget about the real problem which is creating all of this, we'll forget about preventive medicine, and we'll go in and patch things up. We'll be a fix-it man. We're not going to try for something better now, we're just going to stop things up.

Gillian: I don't think Leda's saying that at all. I think she's really putting her mind to what she can do about things practically and immediately. I don't think she's thought about the philosophical area.

Chairman: It's very interesting that Chekhov has picked a man to put the philosophical point of view and a woman to put the practical point of view. What do you think about that?

Nicholas: I think it's a generalization in society that the woman tends to be the more practical, she's expected to do the housework; and the housework of society is to care for the sick and the disabled.

Gillian: I'm not so sure about that, I think it's the man who usually goes out to do things, and it's the woman who frequently has the philosophical approach.

Chairman: What would you say to something that was said to me recently at a gathering: when a man commits himself to exaltation or to self-destruction it's usually over a cause or a principle, but when a woman commits herself to exaltation or to self-destruction it's usually over a person. Second, that there has never been a woman philosopher, mathematician, or musician of note (all disciplines which require a philosophical dimension of thought) and yet in the creative arts of particularity, such as novel writing, women have been every bit as talented as men. It was argued that there was some fundamental difference in the quality of the female mind, compared with the male, and that the female mind naturally moved deductively, that is, from the general to the specific, while the male mind moved inductively from the specific to the general. The male mind was continually moving towards general principles.

Gillian: It's very difficult to know whether, if that habit of thought exists, it's because of the influences which women have been subjected to rather than any fundamental differences between men and women.

Tony: So few women had a university education in the nineteenth century. Women haven't had time to play around with abstract ideas. They just haven't had the opportunity to discuss them in the way one does in the university situation.

David: I think it's a fundamental biological difference, and I don't think it's anything to get uptight about.

Hilary: I don't. I think there's absolutely no difference at all between the minds of men and women. I agree with Gillian.

David: I haven't put a value judgement on which is better. I'm just saying there's a difference. It seems to me a silly thought to deny differences. With such marked physical differences why shouldn't there be some evolutionary intellectual difference?

Nicholas: What a load of rubbish.

David: I resent Nick's comment that my opinion is a load of old rubbish.

Nicholas: Well let me explain. First, I was going to say before that . . .

Chairman [*smiling*]*:* Yes, an uncharacteristic outburst of bad manners, if I might say so Nick.

Nicholas [*ignoring the chairman*]*:* The evidence put forward for a difference in the male and female mind is ridiculous. We've got exceptions on both sides. We've got exceptions proving the rule of millions of people. I don't think you can generalize from highly specialized and creative people to the mass of the people in the population. You're basically making a condemnation of the female mind.

David [*indignantly*]*:* That is an absolute distortion of my point of view. I'm not condemning anything. I don't wish to imply any sort of judgement. Don't talk to me about condemnation.

Nicholas: The reason it's a condemnation is that it makes the statement that there is a biological difference in respect to the human capacities of . . .

David [*interrupting*]*:* Well of course there are biological differences between human beings.

Nicholas: Well I resent that, because *that* has been used as an excuse throughout history for the oppression of people. It *is* a condemnation.

Hilary: I think any apparent differences in the mental approaches between the sexes is just an expression of the repression of woman through the centuries.

Chairman: David, Nicholas's point is that while *you* don't use it as a condemnation, somebody else who is not as altruistic, or as well-balanced, or as kind as you, could use this to 'keep women in their places'.

David: I don't regard a truth as wrong simply because it is used by someone to a bad end. I don't see Wagner's music as bad because the Nazis used it as their theme song.

Chairman: I agree with that to some extent. But if the application of a doctrine invariably produces a bad effect, that does become a criticism. There was a British poet who said, 'What's wrong with Christ is that he was surrounded by a crummy group of advertising managers.'

Rod: Even though his book is still selling!

Chairman: Yes, but I'm eagerly awaiting the next work by the same author before I make up my mind!

Male student: I didn't enjoy it as much as the film!

Jane [*ignoring the jokes*]: I think one helpful bit of evidence in this discussion is that there have been societies in the past where the social roles of men and women have been different and were due to the environment they lived in. In Simone de Beauvour's book, *The Second Sex*, she goes through a history of some early societies which were matriarchal, and where women had the position which men hold today. I don't think anyone's in a position to say what the true potential of women is yet.

Chairman: I suppose it would be a courteous thing to let Jane have the last word today.

Thank you for all your wonderful contributions. You have been an excellent group throughout the whole of the course. Have a good holiday. I hope that as you progress through medical school and your eventual careers the questions and contributions to this course will be remembered.

ESSAY 6

THE PEOPLE AND OUR PROFESSION

There is no life which has not been
determined by a larger public life . . .
and an even larger world of ideas.
George Eliot

The sex and violence in Anthony Burgess's novel, *The Clockwork Orange*, caused a bit of a stir. Perhaps it was essential, either to the purpose of the tale or the sales, to portray in detail Alex's somewhat immoderate behaviour. But it would be a pity if the questions asked by the book and film were left unconsidered by an excited or indignant reader or audience, for some of these questions concern the medical profession.

Doctors do not exist outside the common environment of concepts which influence an age. Indeed, theoretically, no one should be better placed to identify them; for a society is its people, and in dealing with the problems of people in the intense and intimate way which is a doctor's daily task, the rarest of opportunities is available for him to take the pulse of the people and the temperature of their society. With sensitivity and intelligence he can diagnose its deficiency states, its conditions of self-abuse, its excesses, its fears, and its dilemmas. It would be sad if the medical profession stood like an austere bridge beneath whose cold, impassive stones the surge and swell of human frailty flowed, and on whose proud pylons the debris of human suffering washed helplessly before sinking.

In our age there are general attitudes which influence our medical thought and opinion. Our ideas of what is an illness are influenced by these wider concepts; so is our approach to our patients. If our understanding of these concepts is inadequate or inappropriate, our professional ideals and beliefs will also be deficient. When that happens our professional behaviour becomes a little bizarre.

If we could step back from ourselves, we might see more clearly the relevance of our efforts in research and patient care, and our objectives in medical education. When we become aware of the blind spots, astigmatisms, and myopias in our medical vision, our efforts will be better aimed. We might avoid the indignity of appearing to be like those ineffectual scientists met by Gulliver in his travels to Laputa, who busied themselves with the combination and permutation of a few limited concepts. Then we shall look severely at the bias in medicine of superficial symptomatic treatments and turn towards meaningful prevention.

Let us begin by turning our clock back a century. There was a time in the social history of medicine–in the mid-nineteenth century –when public regard for our profession was warm, and when there appeared to be some concord between the ideals of the profession and the public. This affection has been recorded in both literature and personal writings. George Eliot, for example:

> Many of us looking back through life would say the kindest man we have ever known has been a medical man, or perhaps the surgeon whose fine tact, directed by deeply informed perception, has come to us in our need with a more sublime beneficience than that of miracle workers.[1]

Robert Louis Stevenson spoke this praise of doctors:

> The physician is the flower of our civilization; and when that stage of man is done with . . . he will be thought to have shared as little as any of the defects of the period, and most notably exhibited the virtues of the race. Generosity he has, tact, . . . discretion, . . . cheerfulness and courage.[2]

Why was this so? Would we expect to read such professional notices now? I believe the reasons for this affection can be found in a harmony between the performance of the medical profession and the cultural ideals and social interests of Victorian society. As Beatrice Webb observed in her autobiography, *My Apprenticeship:*

> Two outstanding tenets, some would say ideals of the mind, were united in this mid-Victorian trend of thought and feeling. There was the current belief in the scientific method, . . . and the consciousness of a new motive, the transference of the emotion of self-sacrificing service from God to man.[3]

The doctor symbolized these two ideals. In the nineteenth century the doctor was becoming a man of science. His education was pruned of humanities and classics, his amateur researches became more exact and empirical, and his bedside observations were correlated with new theories of aetiology in an attempt to find a cure. Unlike other scientists, the physician met all people and his field had the strongest appeal to laymen. Flaubert, whose father was a doctor, portrayed this enthusiasm in his novel, *Madame Bovary:*

> Honour to these tireless souls who sacrificed their sleep to the advancement of healing of their fellowmen! Honour, thrice honour! Can we not now cry aloud that the blind shall see, the lame walk? But what fanaticism once promised its elect, science now achieves for all mankind![4]

At this time the doctor was seen as a symbol of self-sacrificing service. It was inherent in his work with his readiness to shun concern for personal safety. His duties frequently took him towards danger, into slums, through areas of strife and crime, into epidemics, and into the romantically hard times down crumbling mine shafts. In the nineteenth-century literature, the doctors were seen to turn their backs on 'drawing room values'. Dr Thorne, in a novel of the same name, though a conservative in his beliefs, was odious to one Lady Arabella, says Trollope, 'because of his subversive professional democratic tendencies'. Dr Lydgate, the hero of George Eliot's *Middlemarch*, 'despised any ostentation of exposure; his profession had familiarized him with all grades of poverty and he cared much for those who had suffered hardships.' Both Charles Kingsley and Charles Dickens shared this affection for doctors. Dickens virtually sanctified the medical profession, and had one of his greatest successes as an orator on the profession's behalf when speaking at an appeal for the Great Ormond Street Hospital for Sick Children. Do present-day writers and commentators share this affection for our profession? Are the people today poised ready to applaud?

There were other reasons for public respect and confidence. In the nineteenth century the medical profession became legally defined, registration became necessary, and minimal if not uniform educational standards were gradually established. That mixture of suspect medical degrees which had been referred to by one parliamentarian as 'a parquetry unsafe to walk on' was gradually reinforced by some concrete standards.

The Victorians' secular view of science and sickness also influenced their attitude towards doctors. The belief grew that the onset of disease was avoidable, that technical progress would penetrate its nature and allow pre-symptomatic treatment, and that no disease was incurable. Disease was no longer an agent of God, it was man-made and could be controlled by the doctor. Today we do not have the advantages of this public attitude.

Another factor which raised the standing of the profession one hundred years ago was the great improvement in health produced by the sanitary engineer and the public health doctor. In the nineteenth century, physician reformers such as Sir John Simon and public health legislators like Edwin Chadwick strove to improve the well-being of society and the standards of medicine. They had to overcome professional intransigence and ignorance through education and legislation, and public stupidity through instruction and agitation, aided by the people's fear of epidemics. First through the sanitary engineer, then the medical officer of health—aided by the microscope, the germ theory of disease, and the bacteriological identification of typhoid, cholera, diphtheria, and tuberculosis—the nation was taken from the soap-and-water phase of public health into the scientific. All of these factors contributed to a growing public regard for the nineteenth-century medical profession.

I have generalized for a purpose: to highlight the difference between the public standing of our profession today and that of an earlier generation. Are we still considered special as individuals and noble as a corporate body? Is that earlier regard still justified? Does public trust call for an extraordinary performance and greater responsibility from doctors? And are the present ideas of our age helping or hindering our professional performance?

Some doctors are reassured by commonplace claims such as, 'There is good and bad in everything', or 'Well yes, the *profession* has suffered, but *my* doctor is grand.' As a profession we have a collective responsibility for our own public reputation. We control our profession: we select the original entrants; we teach them by dictate and example; we supervise and judge postgraduate activities; and we set the professional standards. As we exercise these powers, we must be accountable for the quality and integrity of the profession produced. This is what a 'profession' means: we are entrusted with the stewardship of our own standards.

If we believe that the standing of our profession is being undermined, can we identify any of the factors contributing to such a decline?

In an earlier essay I considered the demands of modern doctorship and asked whether they were now beyond the capacity of the average doctor. I asked if modern living and its problems were chewing the juice out of the doctor-patient relationship.

There are different health expectations in different social situations. An impoverished society regards the medical profession as a means to achieve health, whereas an affluent society regards it as a means of obtaining happiness as well as health. This social function of our medical profession shares something not only with the church, but also with alcohol, tobacco, cosmetics, and our various recreational activities. For the most part, in this country, we are dealing with affluent patients.

We are also dealing with patients whose social life is so structured that it contains many pressures forcing them to behave childishly, stupidly, and irresponsibly. Both our religious tradition and our professional ethos support and reinforce the premise that the 'sinful', the weak, and the sick should be helped. Reciprocally, those who exhibit self-reliant behaviour need no help and indeed may be taxed. This rewarding of disability did not apply to the Victorians. It is the undertow created by an attitude which blames parents, society, genes, or what you will, for the blemishes in an individual. It undermines and eventually degrades an individual's sense of personal worth and his personal sense of responsibility. It is a none too subtle form of determinism. And in removing from the patient the consequences of his own irresponsibility in relation to his health, it places an increasing burden on the profession.

I believe the attitude of a society and its serving medical profession towards disease is related to the balance between the material or bodily view of life and the philosophical or spiritual outlook. A materialist society, such as ours, which is concerned with creature comforts, is body-orientated and has no escape from bodily suffering. In such materialist societies which laud the physical, the medical profession has to bear some of the burden of the spiritual void. We do not have the advantages of people in past ages who were assisted through the trials of suffering by their spiritual beliefs:

> Far away is the land of rest,
> Thousand miles are stretched between,
> Many a mountain's stormy crest,
> Many a desert void of green.
>
> Wasted, worn is the traveller;
> Dark his heart and dim his eye;
> Without hope or comforter,
> Faultering, faint, and ready to die . . .
>
> But yet faint not, mournful man;
> Leagues on leagues are left behind
> Since your sunless course began;
> Then go on to toil resigned.
>
> If you still despair control,
> Hush its whispers in your breast,
> You shall reach the final goal,
> You shall win the land of rest.[5]

What of the other influences on our age which affect our professional performance?

I believe much illness is produced by stress, conflict, and the unresolvable human paradoxes. We have allowed the unpleasant aspects of competition to burden those who have been pushed by a policy of mass education, who do not wish to compete, and who feel the stresses of educational and vocational competition. We have allowed technology to intrude into areas of human relationships, displacing the warmth and gentleness of human contact. With the rise of the social sciences and social benefits, we have substituted impersonal corporate handouts for clear interpersonal commitment. In a time of economic nervousness and political anxiety we have subscribed to the goal of short-term gain and gratification, and have sacrificed the ideal of forward planning, for both medical goals and individual aspirations. As professionals who claim increased usefulness as specialists, we have suffered a decline as civilized, cultured citizens.

I agree almost without reservation with the need to uphold the law; for if any of us breaks the law we give equal licence to others, who might not be quite as discerning, to violate laws which are full of sense and stability. But having said that, I am disturbed by the growing obsession with the desire to obey *only* the law, for that creates an attitude of mind in which the law is seen as the only guardian of conduct. So frequently these days one hears the opinion that, provided the law of the land has not been broken, behaviour does not have to be restrained or justified. We hear this sort of talk every day: from the business community, during union disputes, in international or national political arenas, from sportsmen, and from society's numerous sectional associations. We even hear it now from members of our own profession.

This is an attitude which seems to deny the existence of other unwritten codes of conduct, codes such as religious moral convictions, or non-religious principles such as humanism. It dismisses national sentiment, public opinion, local folklore and traditions. It tends to scoff at family loyalties, and at personal conscience. And, most important from our point of view, it undermines professional codes and traditions. Why is this important?

The medical profession, whose unwritten traditions of service and concern are of the greatest importance in maintaining the integrity of its everyday performance, and whose self-monitoring ideals are both precious and delicate, seems particularly vulnerable to the effects of this attitude. The whole of medical practice rests on an unwritten covenant of trust between the doctor and patient. If we are seen to be guiding our actions only by the blunt statutes of the profession or the government, we are in danger of sacrificing what is most valued in our profession. A statement by the Law Society in relation to professional responsibility supports my opinion. 'A professional body', it says, 'should voluntarily submit itself to standards of ethical conduct beyond those required of the ordinary citizens by Law; and secondly, undertake to accept personal responsibility to those whom they serve, and their profession, for maintaining public confidence'.

Now let me move out of the all too bright glare of personal opinion to slide into the shadows of speculation. Let us consider the future. We are now closer to the year 2000 than we are to the year 1950. What will be the position of the medical profession in relation to society fifty years on? I shall not discuss the increasing cost of health, or the progression of 'pill' medicine, for much has already been written and said on the importance of prophylaxis and social medicine.

I believe that over the next half century there will be a gradual increase in government control over individuals, and that before half a century has passed the majority of the peoples of the world (and I include the Western world) will be living under totalitarian controls of either the left wing or the right wing. The movement for greater control will come from the people, at their request, and under their will. Politicians will only reflect the public mood.

Such a state of public detention will arise out of our current social condition and our progressive personal paralysis. We have weakened ourselves to a degree which gives us little protection against the coming man of power. We have become ditherers in our indecision—or even in our concern—about the direction we want the world to take. We are shrivelling in our own apathy. We are slowly becoming disenchanted with social reform, and government handouts. We are unnerved by the economic and political instabilities of our time. We are disenchanted with the ambiguities of judicial decree—our courts' decisions confuse us: the victim is victimized. We can no longer rely on the supply of basic social utilities; and we are vulnerable to the cult of romantic violence. We subscribe to no ordinance beyond man and his worldly preoccupations.

For all these reasons our social priorities will change. 'Necessity,' said Hobbes, 'knows no law.' We are edging towards a state of social disintegration which, when reached, will force us gratefully to donate many of our social freedoms to a power which guarantees the protection of life, property, and creature comforts. Our apathy will be replaced by corporate idealism, and that movement will find its expression in the sanction given to the unhindered power of the state.

In the West we are now facing the last phase in our current cycle of human endeavour. Our human industry is failing—an industry which has passed through a long sequence: proficiency and diligence brought success; this reward caused confidence and familiarity, a liberty which led to improvisation and shortcuts. From there we have suffered a steady decline to negligence and fragmentation. That same sequence which is so frequently followed in a man's life is being mirrored in his social state.

We are no longer bewitched by the variety, the majesty, and the sublimity of things around us. We sit around the stage of life like characters in a Chekhov play, looking for trivial pursuits to relieve our chronic boredom. Never before have so many done so little, with such gracelessness, and at such expense, under the name of leisure and recreation.

Democracy is not a rigid system, nor an implacable doctrine. It is an attitude of mind—a habit of conduct. We are gradually losing our tolerance for the extravagances of egalitarianism. Circumstances will soon show that such tolerance is too expensive both politically and socially; and, as it is circumstances which render civil schemes beneficial or noxious to mankind, many of our indulgent freedoms will be considered luxuries. Individualism will then suffer and be forced into a private underground: a resistance movement of the spirit.

I have put forward this extreme and perhaps aberrant position for a purpose: to ask what has this to do with the medical profession? If it is untrue–nothing. The unlimited resources of human ingenuity, creativity, and imagination, and the human desire to breathe, will guarantee that if such a movement came, it would be short lived. Human beings love to dance, and the other great force gradually coming to the social surface–the rise of the irrational–will guarantee a lot of dancing in the middle of the next century.

But if there is some small truth in my theoretical proposition then the importance could be profound.

First, such a government might introduce a system of personal accountability for sickness. That is to say, to the extent that an individual was responsible for his disease, he would be penalized. In the extreme, a patient whose disease was produced by personal folly (alcohol, cigarettes, overeating, self-induced stress, drugs, careless driving) would simply be refused treatment. A government which was concerned only with efficiency would not be concerned about personal needs, particularly if those indulgences were an unproductive drain on social resources. This Erewhonian system of social justice would force the individual to confront himself with the consequences of his own actions.

Second, medicine would be such an important potential weapon in the hands of a despotic power, that the profession is sure to be first courted, then–if it is refractory–clubbed, by such a power. This was the medical message in *The Clockwork Orange*.

In such a tyrannical state, doctors may be ordered to work under direct state control and dictate. They may be recruited as agents or arms of government policy, and asked to work for the dubious or overtly evil physical or psychological ends of the controlling power. In view of the apparently natural right-wing sentiments of our profession, I fear we are probably more likely to be urged into acts of ethical ambiguity on behalf of a right-wing government. As I mentioned in the last session, during the early 1950s meetings were held in our medical community to decide if doctors should reveal the political sentiments of some of their left-wing patients to the government.

Any government intrusion of this sort is alien to medical practice as we now cherish it. Government dictate, or even government legislation, is incapable of assessing and allowing for the many human immeasurables which are part of the clinical landscape. This is one of the inherent deficiencies of law. This is why Dickens called the law 'a ass'.[6]

Perhaps all this is a speculative aberration. Perhaps the medical profession will be able to stand aside from severe political movements and gaze on them with indifference and detachment. But before we reach that cosy conclusion let us consider this paragraph from the preface Aldous Huxley wrote for his novel, *Brave New World* (a novel originally banned in Australia), and note two things: how much the medical profession is involved in his prophetic prescription, and–what is more important–how much more capable we are likely to be in the future of presenting a political power with the sort of ammunition he outlines.

> The love of servitude cannot be established except as the result of a deep, personal revolution in human minds and bodies. To bring about that revolution we require, among others, the following discoveries and inventions. First, a greatly improved technique of suggestion–through infant conditioning and, later, with the aid of drugs, such as scopolamine. Second, a fully developed science of human differences, enabling government managers to assign any given individual to his or her proper place in the social and economic hierarchy. (Round pegs in square holes tend to have dangerous thoughts about the social system and to infect others with their discontents.) Third (since reality, however utopian, is something from which people feel the need of taking pretty frequent holidays), a substitute for alcohol and the other narcotics, something at once less harmful and more pleasure-giving than gin or heroin. And fourth (but this would be long-term project, which would take generations of totalitarian control to bring to a successful conclusion), a foolproof system of eugenics, designed to standardize human product and so to facilitate the task of the managers. In *Brave New World* this standardization of the human product has been pushed to fantastic, though not perhaps impossible, extremes.[7]

We have only one protection against such a political movement. A complete dedication to the principle of individualism and individual creativity. Not the sort of invalid individualism which is sliding us towards the condition of apathy and inertia, and which will produce total vulnerability. But the vigorous individualism of agitated, restless, and irreverent people who ripple with ideas and interests, and who subscribe to self-realization before state subservience:

> A human being is a member of the community, not as a limb is a member of a body . . . intended only to contribute to some joint result. He is an ultimate being made for his own perfection and his higher end, made to maintain an individual existence and to serve others only as far as consists with his own virtue and progress.[8]

The religion of individuality is the only possible protection against totalitarianism; and the qualities of self which are dominant in that defence are creativity and imagination.

We should try to give scope to the creative mind. We must seek it out, foster and protect it. Creativity should be the first object of worship in a secular society. We must try to create the conditions necessary for its growth; and acknowledge to ourselves that its richest gifts and choicest products will often be beyond our commonplace understanding.

Perhaps there is an irony when one who begs and borrows from other creative minds runs a crusade for creativity. I admit my piracy with the excuse that my borrowings have been as the bee's: I have tried to absorb the sweet offerings of others in an attempt to produce some small nectar of my own. Just as a man with one leg can tell you how important it is to have two limbs to climb, I plead for the conditions that cultivate creativity, without being able to demonstrate such fruits of my own.

COMMENTS ON THE COURSE

Rod

Although I entered the seminar room rather sceptically the first afternoon, I found this course very beneficial. I felt it broadened my medical learning experience by helping to fill areas which had been seriously neglected in our course so far–interpersonal communication, both verbal and, especially non-verbal. It has made me more aware of the problems and pitfalls that a doctor faces in his dealings with patients, their relatives, the public, and even fellow doctors. I hope I shall be better able to avoid, or at least cope with them.

David

The six weeks of this course have been a uniquely enjoyable and stimulating experience in my medical education. I feel that in scientific courses generally there is far too little consideration of the vast range of human cultural achievement. In medicine especially, consideration of literature, art, music, etc. provides an enriching experience which can only be of benefit to the individual concerned. A medical course should be seen as an education in the broadest sense, rather than an exercise in fact accumulation.

The other excellent aspect of the course was that it provided a forum for discussion of aspects of medicine not normally covered in most formal teaching sessions, where the emphasis is on diagnosis and treatment of illness, rather than the broader issues of patient-doctor relationships, professional attitudes, and the personal (as opposed to the physical) aspects of the patient's condition. This course is an exciting innovation, which should be continued, and expanded.

Gillian

I think that during the medical humanities sessions, some of us in the group said more to each other then we had in the last four years of medicine–and discovered that we actually did have something in common after all! The fact that every student was present at the final session–which happened to be on the last day of the year, when all self-respecting medical students would normally be down at the pub–gives a good indication of our appreciation of the course.

Nicholas

One of the greatest fears in my life is that I might become an insular, undirectional automaton. I've always tried to have multiple commitments of a significant kind, i.e. other than just job and leisure. Thus one reason for my emotional embracement of the experience of this course is that it has rekindled something which I enjoyed during school but which I've had to neglect due to pressures of university commitments–political and academic. For this selfish reason I found the experience invaluable.

Apart from this, there is, of course, the essential educational benefit, specifically my exposure to a rich spectrum of human experience in the medical context. Especially valuable were the sessions where the commonest (but also the most disregarded) medical situations were presented in the context of their full significance and complexity from a particular viewpoint.

But I maintain some reservations (and perhaps these belong in the assessment questionnaire rather than here). The discussions springing from consideration of the presented material were sometimes frightening. Usually they were based on political, moral, and ethical opinions and anecdotal prejudices–rather than sociological, psychiatric, and epidemiological information. When a statement is made, e.g. 'Most patients don't wish to know they are dying' or 'Women prefer female doctors', the time is highly appropriate for presentation of data. All such statements should be clearly indicated by the moderator as generalizations which require statistical support, which may or may not exist, but is not available during the current discussion. Debates based on groundless suppositions are especially dangerous in the medical (? objective) context since they merely reinforce prejudices.

Discussions involving basic principles, moral and political, are invaluable in clarifying motivation for thought and action. Indeed, this is where the 'participator' aspect of the course flourishes. There is vast difference between a discussion on 'Most patients *should* be told they are dying' and 'Most patients don't want to be told they are dying'–although having said that I already see a grey zone–so I offer no solutions.

During such discussions, trying to evolve a consensus among the group sometimes seems an intrusion on individuality. 'Professional solidarity', an infinitely arguable concept in itself, should not be a blanketing device to resolve chasms of moral difference.

Again I wish to reiterate the value of this course, perhaps, on reflection, even more valuable for *me* with its deficiencies intact. Thank you.

Colin

The main reasons why the course was beneficial are as follows.

It allowed a more formal arena for discussion of problems we experience as students and doctors in our relationships with others outside the medical community: for example, feelings of alienation and suspicion, and an unwarranted faith in us by patients, or other feelings of desperate dependence on us by our patients. The reasons why these exist were discussed, and how to deal with them was tackled in the forum.

It reinforced or awakened an awareness in the students of the difficulties and problems faced by patients and relatives. A need for total patient appraisal was emphasized, one which included not only the patient and his medical condition, but the reactions of the family, relatives, and community; also the patient's wishes during his life and the prejudices of those treating him.

The course was fun. It was evident Dr Moore was enjoying this new adventure and relating to students in the different way the forum allowed. The literature was relevant and of a type (wider-ranging though it was) that I like.

Brendan

I feel that this course, although it has not changed my basic ideas, has given me an opportunity to greatly clarify my somewhat nebulous thoughts about many of the human aspects of medicine—by virtue of the fact that I have been 'forced' to express an opinion on the specific issues which were raised. It has also given me a large amount of insight into many of my fellow students, and, to a certain extent, has stimulated discussion between students on issues which were previously only rarely brought up.

Hilary

This exercise in medical humanities has for me been the most valuable single segment of the medical course so far, being both enjoyable purely as a study of literature, and worthwhile in the context of training to practise medicine.

Having always had a special interest in English literature I was unhappy to relinquish such studies when deprived of the opportunity within the medical curriculum. It seems that the need to encompass an enormous range of disciplines within the strict confines of medicine allows no time for a broader education to continue. Apparently, by definition, a study of medicine precludes perusal of any other academic interest.

Therefore these sessions have been a welcome relief: a refreshing Friday afternoon eagerly awaited each week. Compared with schoolday literature classes, the appreciation has increased, as passages are viewed now with a greater maturity than that enjoyed by a school child. The large amount of time spent, by necessity, in clinical work also adds to the appreciation of a few short hours of humanities.

More importantly, the exercise was of great value in training for doctorship, because of the relevance of the subject material considered. The issues forming the basis of the discussions are ones which should be considered vital to the practice of good medicine and which have been too long neglected. Clinicians, in their desire to impart maximum knowledge to their students, forget the interpersonal relationships involved in doctoring, and the basic need for communication. This course, in bringing such aspects to our attention, is beginning to compensate for a hitherto abysmal lack. What use is the ability to recite every textbook ever written, without the ability to develop at least an adequate doctor-patient relationship, and understand how the patient may feel?

The format based on discussion amongst students was ideal, allowing us to think, formulate ideas, and communicate with each other. We have not had many such opportunities to express ourselves. Each student had much to offer, and much to learn from the others.

There will be, I am sure, a long-term benefit, as we take an altered outlook back to the wards, and continue to consider points raised at these sessions.

Finally, I wish to express how privileged I feel to have taken part in this course, and to say thank you.

Dave

I enjoyed the course but found that some of the discussions were a little out of line as far as providing an opportunity for extracting a conclusion from them. I know I went away from some with little realization of how I can relate my personality to my medical practice. Indeed, some of the discussions, paragraphs, and extracts were more like an English lesson, than a discussion which is relevant to us as future doctors. That is what the course should be more aimed at.

Robert

Dr Moore's sessions provided the students with a regular forum for discussion. Although there was a set topic for discussion each week the course was not narrow or limited; each topic was broad enough in itself to allow a wide range of argument. When I started the course I thought it would be a boring Friday afternoon; however, with the exception of a few minor dull periods, the sessions were most interesting. Not only did I think about my views, but I learned how the other members of the group thought, how they approached a problem, and in some cases how easily they were upset by a bit of gentle prodding. The course was interesting and well worth while. I hope in future years it can be greatly expanded, not only in fourth year but into other years as well.

Stuart

I found the medical humanities sessions a pleasant break from the didactic atmosphere of the fourth-year course. Unfortunately they were not as slack as I had anticipated and in fact produced an intense involvement from all the students. I appreciated the chance to exchange views on the less easily defined aspects of medicine and its relation to the community. The use of selected literature was a cunning method of introducing topics for discussion.

I have always felt that there should be more room in the course for the study of humanities and Dr Moore's sessions are a very practical start.

Tony

In the clinical years of a medical course it is so very easy to neglect ourselves as complete personalities. Heavy workloads and the pressure to appreciate primarily the physical basis of clinical problems tend to engender an attitude of callous disregard for patients as people.

Medical humanities provided an opportunity for us both to formulate a broader view of medical practice and to discuss and develop more personal issues in an informal atmosphere. In this respect it satisfied two major deficiencies of medical education, namely the absence of any social and cultural perspective, and the lack of opportunity for students to express individual viewpoints, particularly on ethical questions.

The use of extracts from works of literature and philosophy as the basis for discussions contributed substantially to the success of the course. Vivid literary portrayals of illness, despair, medical arrogance and ineptitude, and patient dependence stimulated vigorous and animated exchanges, rarely full agreement; and for all of us a classification and consolidation of viewpoints on probably the most important questions arising in a medical career.

Doug

I doubt whether the following comments are of significance as I unavoidably missed two of the Friday afternoon sessions, and I have never been of a literary inclination, so I am afraid my view may well appear simplistic.

Overall I found the sessions a great relief from the hospital rat-race by providing a perspective of the atmosphere in which the physician and surgeon live and work, and the degrees of respect in which they have been held. It certainly suppresses any sense of superiority which could emerge after spending several years on the medical scene and being accorded the respect of an elite club.

As regards the course, I was more than impressed with the visual side [slides of paintings], mainly because, I suppose, my artistic background is virtually non-existent. I found it most interesting and stimulating. The poetry and literary extracts often did not make an impression on me, usually due to the antiquated style of writing which I found required considerable concentration, and sometimes caused confusion. However certain pieces were highly eloquent, even to my inexperienced self. Samuel Johnson's poem and Shakespeare's poems were especially impressive and it was these (and a few other small extracts) which I was interested enough to read over again at home.

I suppose I often appeared rather distant in many of the discussions, not through any lack of interest, but rather in deep thought as I feel I was often slow to grasp the significance of many passages. I must admit that in all my schooling I had never gained such a deep insight into poetry and English literary extracts as I gained in these sessions. I guess it's a sign of maturity, as such material, if presented to me while at high school, would have been ridiculed.

Jane

The six sessions of medical humanities helped to fill a very wide gap which exists in the present medical course.

The structure of the medical course is extremely restrictive. Original thought and non-establishment points of view are frowned upon. No time is given for the consideration of the complications of being a doctor–moral, social, and political issues are virtually never discussed except by the occasional enlightened tutor. The social relationships between patients and doctors are rarely touched upon. Such a situation leads to the production of doctors who know textbook descriptions of diseases word for word, but who have no concept of relating in any meaningful way to the people they treat. The structure of the medical course is designed to perpetuate a conservative profession completely isolated from the people it should be serving.

Medical humanities was a welcome addition to the medical course. If the idea is extended it has the potential to change the present situation. An ideal course would provide a forum for free discussions of the issues mentioned above, which are currently suppressed, as well as bringing students into wider contact with the arts.

Liz

I found the medical humanities course interesting and stimulating. I think that perhaps it was most helpful in that it enabled me to hear the views of other students on the issues discussed. Often we tend to believe that the majority of our contemporaries necessarily have similar views on most issues. I was consequently enlightened by the diversification of opinions that were frequently apparent.

It also provided a stimulus for me to examine my own attitudes, many of which were clarified during the course of the discussions.

The choice of the literature was, I thought, generally suitable, but I felt that some of the passages were somewhat obscure and unnecessary.

Overall, I enjoyed the Friday afternoon sessions and I really do believe that they have made some contribution to my awareness of the attitudes I have, relevant to being involved in the medical profession.

I thank you for taking the trouble to organize the experiment and wish you success in its further progress which will inevitably be the case.

Chairman and Author

These sessions show that medical students have strong views on many important medical topics. Some expressed indignation over the decline in our professional distinction and public regard. Others are concerned about the need to protect the delicacies of the doctor-patient relationship from both crass government intrusion, and our professional stubbornness. Almost all acknowledged a belief in the unique privileges and pressures of being a member of the medical guild.

To those who are familiar with the concepts we have discussed and who already practise the alternatives explored, I can only offer my admiration, and add a word of gratitude. You are the living example of what we have tried to capture on the page: you already practise what we have tried to plead. Most of what we have said is simple.

Speaking personally, I have not written this book to put everything in the profession right, but to make what's wrong as little as possible; for while we as humans have imperfections, so shall our systems. Nor am I writing to challenge the old dogmas of the profession with an offering of some new ones—there is little merit in replacing a rusty chain with a polished one. I wish to support the spirit which questions all dogma. In our attempt to see the problems before us we have stood on the shoulders of thinkers of ages past. I must confess my waywardness: I have borrowed greatly from minds of other writers to apply their insights to the medical profession. My plagiaristic habit has been eccentric but well-intentioned, for, as in one and the same field the cow looks for grass, the fox for the hare, and the hawk for the vulnerable, I, in their plots, have searched for a way of saying. Nor can I atone for misuse of their works by giving them adequate acknowledgment.

This book is concerned with medical reform. In this last comment I would like to explore some of the problems involved with trying to change medical habits.

When a foot becomes gangrenous one doesn't hobble along praising its 'sometime swiftness'. As a profession we seem to be in danger of imprisoning ourselves by the lines we have drawn in order to exclude the concepts of others outside our ranks. The medical humanities course is an attempt to expand the short spectrum of our medical studies with medically relevant extracts from literary works. It tries to do something new.

I have no affection for the 'established' just for its own sake. Yet I have no inclination to embrace changes which produce only immediate gratification. It seems to me important to distinguish between what is established to be right, and what is right because it is established. What we call necessary institutions are often no more than institutions to which we have grown accustomed. But it is the elders who control the policies in our profession, and it is difficult for old men to change; they usually bring about change by guiding and guarding the opportunities of the young who have the drive and desire to initiate change. The task of changing attitudes is not easy. As Doctor Johnson noted in his life of Milton, 'Every man that has ever undertaken to instruct others, can tell what slow advances he has been able to make, and how much patience it requires to reach even vagrant inattention, to stimulate sluggish indifference, and to rectify absurd misapprehension.'

Our profession *is* conservative, but one cannot stand forever on a branch one is sawing through. The conservatism of our profession has many elements and expressions, and it is important that we understand them all before we decide our preference between progress and preservation; for they will influence our ability to initiate reforms.

First, there is practical conservatism, or that simple and sensible caution which denies any new theory or therapy until it has been tested for any sinister or unsuspected side-effects. Whereas it is true that each medical prescription is an experiment, it should be one in which the patient has been offered the safest and soundest therapeutic chance. No one disagrees with this.

The second is what I call traditionalist conservatism: an attitude of mind which has an affection for the heritage of the profession, and which respects the order that has been slowly developed through the composite wisdom of its members. It is an attitude which grows out of a knowledge of the history of medicine as described both in standard source books and in the popular literature and letters of a period. It shows a respect for the evolution of the profession's educational and ethical standards, for the medical fraternity, and for the tradition of mutual support for members who are inexperienced, unwell, or upset. Critics of traditionalist conservatism say that those who embrace it confuse the satisfaction gained at giving an explanation of a situation with satisfaction at the situation. But that is unfair. Rather I would say they are aware that it is easier to overturn something than to support it. The world can be toppled with the tip of a finger on a lever, but it needs the shoulders of Atlas to support it. I believe traditionalist conservatism is the only outlook which is compatible with an awareness of one's cultural heritage, and with a desire for the preservation of influences and traditions which have given stability, dignity, and moderation to life. This is not just my view. It is part of human nature's mass sentiment. Time as well as truth is needed to overcome tradition. This is not to say that elements in a society or profession should not be subject to scrutiny and change.

It is reactionary conservatism which opposes change. This is an attitude which unfortunately intrudes frequently into our profession. It is both unacceptable and dangerous for it is commonly set down by those with mediocre minds. There are some who seem to have an affection for the artificial stability produced by an inflexible rule. They feel no wonder and ask no questions about what is constantly before their eyes. For them, it is familiarity rather than conviction which accounts for most beliefs. They wish to establish the sort of stability in which we can all perish safely. The opinions of an authority they often confuse with the 'laws of nature'. If one was kind, one would say that they are not so much blind as blinkered, not mistaken so much as misled. I believe that every profession is perpetually degenerating towards settled opinions. It accepts revered beliefs from which it must be rescued at certain periods by the resuscitation of its first principles, and by the re-establishment of its original ideals. Now while I know that the views and opinions of the profession have not evolved without thought and assessment, and that for the most part they are successful, powerful, and worthy of respect, I also feel that there arrive periods when circumstances and conditions have changed, and that the guiding rules of the profession ought to change also.

Conservatism should not mean intransigence and ossification; it has always pleaded for a broad view and has always tried to relate new happenings to historical events. One can be a reformer yet a conservative, for if one believes in the importance of proportion and harmony then one is always trying to reform a state of imbalance, be it in one's life, one's society, or one's profession.

A conservative medical reformer today may be trying to alter the imbalance in the criteria on which medical students are selected; the exclusivity of scientism in their studies; the lack of adequate opportunity to discuss the human problems of disease; or the exclusivity of hospital-orientated teaching. The issues will alter with the age. But the principle remains: deficiencies must be made up, excesses amputated. This book has been motivated by that principle.

And yet, even with the issues defined, our profession is slow to reform itself. This is especially so in the area of social medicine. In part, this is due to our *political* conservatism. I believe the medical school curricula should offer the opportunity to discuss the problem of the disproportionate political representation in our profession and how it affects our relationship with governments–particularly socialist governments–on matters of medico-political importance. How much do doctors know about the cost distribution of the health bill? And how much do they know about the distribution and utilization of hospital health services, or public health services?

The university has a central position in relation to medical reform. As student members of the medical profession we sometimes forget that we are also members of a university community. Although the institutional ideals of the profession and the academy overlap, they are not identical. It is the universities which should generate change.

I believe that a university is a special place which has a unique function and purpose in society. Its staff members are protected in their jobs by tenure of appointment. This concept (despite the popular belief that the term now means only guaranteed job security) was originally designed to protect an academic's freedom to speak out on any issue–political, social, religious, or moral. That is, it was designed to protect what I cherish as the essence of what it means to be an academic: it allows total critical questioning on all subjects. It permits a healthy irreverence towards prevailing beliefs, methods, and mores. It stimulates a full exploration of the cultural significance and intellectual tradition of one's field of study. And it should promote in students, by example, the quality of critical judgement.

A university has a paradoxical relationship with truth: it is its guardian and its assassin; it protects a standing truth, yet it is trying incessantly to replace it. Nothing can be spared from this intellectual provocation and attack. The only profanity in a university is stasis. Rigidity, cosiness, contentment, and immutability, are the enemies against which academics must always agitate. Tension between the conservative medical profession and a healthy university is therefore inevitable.

Our noble profession has an ignoble talent for self-deception. We have in our ranks many who wish to wear the clothes of the emperor, and too few who stand up and suggest he is without them. We tend to deceive ourselves about the disparity between our professional disputes and our professional dignity; between therapeutic claim and therapeutic cure; between prescribing and prophylaxis; and between the concern for pay and the concern for patients. The margin between status and service is blurred. These are all examples of aberrations of our professional ideal–aberrations that we seem tacitly to deny. This professional self-contentment rests uneasily beside the tradition of restless academic agitation that is the feature of all flourishing universities.

Another attitude that hinders reform is that the public, the politicians, and even the profession, all expect that the work of the medical faculty should be heavily practical. That is to say, *all* our activities–our research and thought, our time and teaching, and our clinical care–should be directed and expressed in terms of our service component. The concept of medical scholarship for scholarship's sake is thought of as a meaningless void. Aspects of medical scholarship such as medical philosophy, social concepts of disease, the relationship of medicine to government or society, and the interaction between medicine and social history or the history of ideas, are almost totally ignored. This attitude is even spreading into the universities themselves. Specialist faculties do not tolerate generalist projects.

If this is true, and I feel sadly that it is, we should all recommend that medical faculties, with their apparent intolerance of the spirit of unfettered scholarship, change their names to 'medical technical college' or 'college of domestic medical science'.

The true spirit of scholarship is not subservient to utilitarian requirements, or to professional conservatism–it stands aside from both, and regards them with some indifference. If usefulness is made the ultimate arbiter of academic worth, common opinions and needs will determine the direction of scholarship. And the most massive danger of this is that the common mind then determines the scope of scholarship. This is absolutely unacceptable. For it is in the nature of the products of the uncommon mind–those thoughts and discoveries which add new frames to the structure of truth–that they cannot be anticipated, and that they are frequently misunderstood or unintelligible to those of us who measure all by what is known, or common, or useful.

In part, I believe governments have been responsible for the emasculation of the academy. They have accepted the economic responsibilities of intellectual and creative patronage, while at the same time they have superimposed controls on the direction of scholarship. They have assumed that as the public pays for universities, the public must have some obvious and immediate benefit. I believe that when social utility becomes the guardian of scholarship, excellence is sacrificed for advantage. It is during times of greatest economic or political stress, such as in our present day, that the ideals of the university are threatened and in need of greatest protection. A social history of medicine has never been prepared as an academic study; nor has a work tracing the development of professional attitudes in medicine; nor a work relating the history of medicine to the general history of ideas. Each of them would require a special individual who has remained independent of the profession's current preoccupations. It is individuals who initiate change.

The wit of George Bernard Shaw once quipped that the doctor who gets ahead of his patients' prejudices is a ruined man. Had he been a member of our guild he might have made the slightly shrewder observation that the same fate awaits a doctor who gets ahead of his profession's customs.

There is little doubt that the medical apprenticeship tends to straighten the natural crooked line of individual personality, and tends to replace it, at least in a professional context, with a corporate personality. People at parties can usually discover a doctor, for there is something of a sameness about them. They share a professional personality which brings both benefits and liabilities.

Uniformity arouses a combative spirit because–to use Charles Darwin's phrase–'competition is greatest between those who occupy the same position in the economy of nature'. Similarity produces like needs and desires; individualism, by its very nature, has divergent desires. Competition is an ambiguous human quality, for though it can stimulate excellence, achievement, and even comradeship amongst talented people, it can also reveal pettiness, ruthlessness, and mean-mindedness in those who are mediocre. One of the dangers of professional uniformity and conformity is that free expression of specific individual talents is thwarted, and all the adverse effects of competition are encouraged. The trouble with clambering up ladders is that one's backside is exposed, and that upon the most exalted throne in the world we still have to sit on our bottoms. Unfortunately, students are shown many examples of the sort of ambition which walks on tip-toes or goes on all fours. Most of them are aware, however, that one is unstable and the other undignified. Devotion to competition against others undermines individuality.

The ideal of individualism has been the conscience of this book: the individuality of all patients, nurses, doctors, and students.

Through the course I have come to know Tony's sensitivity, Jane's humanity, Brendan's wisdom, Dave's kind nature, Doug's humility, Stuart's desire to doubt, Robert's humour, Colin's well-balanced sense, Rod's quickness of mind, Hilary's intelligence, Nicholas's idealism, Gillian's honesty, David's application, and Liz's common sense.

NOTES

THE ART OF MEDICINE

[1] This essay is based on my article "The Art of Medicine: A Missing Subject?", which appeared in the *Medical Journal of Australia* (1975), vol. 2, pp. 27-8

[2] George Eliot, *Middlemarch* (1871-2), ch. 15.

[3] A. Chekhov, 'A Boring Story', in *Lady with Lapdog and Other Stories*, trans. David Magarshack (Harmondsworth, Mddx, 1964).

[4] Charles Kingsley, *Two Years Ago* (1856), ch. 5.

[5] F. H. Garrison, *An Introduction to the History of Medicine*, 4th ed. (London and Philadelphia, 1929), p. 883.

[6] W. Osler in *Montreal Medical Journal* (1897), vol. 26, p. 186.

[7] Matthew Arnold, *Discourses in America* (London and New York, 1889), pp. 78-9.

[8] Quoted in *ibid.*, p. 98.

[9] J. W. Goethe, *Elective Affinities* (1808), trans. J. A. Froude (London, 1901), pt 2, ch. 3.

[10] P. B. Shelley, *The Letters of Percy Bysshe Shelley*, ed. Roger Ingpen (London, 1909), vol. 1, p. 75.

THE MEDICAL HUMANITIES COURSE

[1] A. Gregg, 'Humanism and Science', *Bulletin of the New York Academy of Medicine* (February 1941), pp. 94-5.

SESSION 1

[1] A. Solzhenitsyn, *Cancer Ward*, trans. Nicholas Bethell and David Burg (Harmondsworth, Mddx, 1968), ch. 2.

[2] Sylvia Plath, *The Bell Jar* (1963), p. 68.

[3] Charles Lamb, 'The Convalescent', in *Last Essays of Elia* (1829-33).

[4] Virginia Woolf, 'On Being Ill', in *The Moment and Other Essays* (London, 1947).

[5] André Gide, *The Immoralist* (1902), trans. Dorothy Bussy (Harmondsworth, Mddx, 1973), ch. 6.

[6] Gwen Wesson, *Brian's Wife, Jenny's Mum* (Melbourne, 1975), pp. 19-21.

[7] Elizabeth Gaskell, *Mary Barton* (1848), ch. 15.

ESSAY 1

[1] S. Garth, 'The Dispensary' (1669), canto 1, in *British Poets*, ed. Park, vol. 9 (London, 1808).

[2] Thomas Mann, *The Magic Mountain* (1924), trans. H. T. Lowe-Porter (Harmondsworth, Mddx, 1973), chs 4, 5.

[3] J. Cocteau, *Les Enfants Terribles*, trans. Rosemary Lehmann (Harmondsworth, Mddx, 1973), p. 139.

[4] Seneca, *Epistulae Morales ad Lucilium* (62-5 A.D.), trans. Robin Campbell as *Letters from a Stoic* (Harmondsworth, Mddx, 1974), letter XCI, pp. 178-9.
[5] Ibid., p. 181.
[6] Leo Tolstoy, *War and Peace* (1868-9), trans. Louise and Aylmer Maude (World's Classics, London, 1958), bk 11, ch. 32.
[7] Mann, *op. cit.*, ch. 4.

SESSION 2

[1] Theodore Dreiser, 'The Lost Phoebe', in *The Best Short Stories of Theodore Dreiser* (1947).
[2] L. Rinser, 'An Old Man Dies', trans. Arthur S. Wensinger, quoted in *The Abnormal Personality Through Literature*, A. A. Stone and S. S. Stone (eds), (Prentice-Hall Inc., New Jersey, 1966).
[3] W. Shakespeare, Sonnet 66 (c. 1590).
[4] Enid Blyton, *The Magic Faraway Tree* (London, 1940), ch. 20.
[5] Conrad Aiken, 'Silent Snow, Secret Snow', in *Collected Short Stories of Conrad Aiken* (1932).
[6] Gillian Coote, 'My Grandmother in the Shower', in Kate Jennings (ed.), *Mother I'm Rooted* (Melbourne, 1975).

ESSAY 2

[1] This essay is based on my article 'A Medical Message from Literature', which appeared in *Surgery, Gynecology and Obstetrics* (1977), vol. 145, pp. 90-3, and is reprinted by permission.
[2] W. Shakespeare, *King Lear* (1606), act III, sc. vi.
[3] P. B. Shelley, 'A Defence of Poetry', in *The Prose of Percy Bysshe Shelley*, ed. Roger Ingpen (London, 1909), vol. 7, p. 118.
[4] George Eliot, quoted in John W. Cross, *George Eliot's Life* (London, 1885), vol. 2, p. 118.
[5] J. W. Goethe, *Elective Affinities* (1808), trans. J. A. Froude (London, 1901), p. 141.
[6] Charles Lamb, 'In Praise of Chimney Sweepers', in *Essays of Elia* (1820-33).
[7] H. F. Amiel, *Fragments D'un Journal Intime* (1883), quoted in R. M. Magraw, *Ferment in Medicine* (Saunders, U.S.A., 1966), p. 15.
[8] John Aubrey, 'William Harvey', in *Brief Lives* (1650-97).
[9] W. Shakespeare, *Hamlet* (1605), act I, sc. ii.
[10] II Samuel xiv. 34.

SESSION 3

[1] Sinclair Lewis, *Arrowsmith* (1924), ch. 11.
[2] A. Chekhov, 'A Boring Story', in *Lady with Lapdog and Other Stories*, trans. David Magarshack (Harmondsworth, Mddx, 1964).
[3] Charles Lamb, 'Imperfect Sympathies', in *Essays of Elia* (1820-33).
[4] Simone de Beauvoir, *A Very Easy Death*, trans. Patrick O'Brian (Harmondsworth, Mddx, 1976).
[5] Somerset Maugham, *Of Human Bondage* (1915), ch. 81.
[6] Samuel Johnson, 'On the Death of Dr Robert Levet' (1760).
[7] George Crabbe, *The Village* (1783), bk 1.
[8] A. J. Cronin, *The Citadel* (1937), pt 1, ch. 7; pt 4, ch. 4.
[9] J. Brown, 'Rab and his Friends', in *Horae Subsecivae* (Edinburgh, 1882), vol. 2, p. 377.
[10] Thomas Mann, *The Magic Mountain* (1924), trans. H. T. Lowe-Porter (Harmondsworth, Mddx, 1973), ch. 5.

ESSAY 3

[1] W. Shakespeare, *Julius Caesar* (1599), act IV, sc, iii.
[2] Thomas Carlyle, *Sartor Resartus* (1831), bk 2, ch. 7.
[3] Robert Browning, 'Andrea del Sarto' (1885).
[4] A. Conan-Doyle, 'A Medical Document', in *Round the Red Lamp* (London, 1894).
[5] Nathaniel Hawthorne, *The Scarlet Letter* (1850), ch. 9.
[6] George Crabbe, *The Borough* (1810), letter 3.
[7] A. Conan-Doyle, 'Behind the Times', in *op. cit.*

SESSION 4

[1] C. P. Snow, *The Masters* (London, 1951), chs 1-3.
[2] A. R. Moore, 'Truth and Consent', in *Medical Journal of Australia* (1977), vol. 1, pp. 451-4.
[3] *Age* (Melbourne), 26 October 1976.
[4] Moore, *op. cit.*
[5] Nathaniel Hawthorne, *The Scarlet Letter* (1850), ch. 9.
[6] B. de Mandeville, *The Fable of the Bees* (1714), remark P.
[7] H. G. Wells, *The Island of Dr Moreau* (1896), ch. 14.
[8] G. B. Shaw, *Doctor's Dilemma* (1906), p. lxiii.

ESSAY 4

[1] This essay is based on my article 'Truth and Consent', which appeared in the *Medical Journal of Australia* (1977), vol. 1, pp. 451-4.
[2] R. W. Emerson, 'Experience' (1844), in *Essays* (Everyman, London, 1971).
[3] 'Report of Medical Ethics: Canada', in *World Medical Association Bulletin* (1949), vol. 1, no. 3, p. 109.
[4] P. Ramsey, *Patient as Person* (Yale, 1970), p.xv.

SESSION 5

[1] Virginia Woolf, *Mrs Dalloway* (1926), pp. 100-2.
[2] *Ibid.*, pp. 105-10.
[3] A. Brownjohn, 'For a Journey', in *Penguin Modern Poets no. 14* (Harmondsworth, Mddx, 1969).
[4] Lewis Carroll, *Through the Looking Glass* (1872), ch. 6.
[5] Virginia Woolf, 'On Being Ill', in *The Moment and Other Essays* (London, 1947).
[6] James Joyce, *A Portrait of the Artist as a Young Man* (1916), ch. 5.
[7] D. H. Lawrence, *Sons and Lovers* (1913), ch. 14.
[8] Henry James, *The Wings of the Dove* (1902), ch. 12.

ESSAY 5

[1] A. Pope, 'Moral Essays: Epistle to Cobham', ll. 101-2, in *The Poems of Alexander Pope*, ed. J. Butt (London, 1970).
[2] Emile Zola, quoted in Leo Tolstoy, 'Non-Acting', in *Recollections and Essays*, trans. Aylmer Maude (World's Classics, London, 1961).
[3] *Ibid.*

SESSION 6

[1] Parliamentary Act of 1511, quoted in Sir George Clarke, *A History of the Royal College of Physicians of London* (Oxford, 1964), vol. 1, ch. 4.
[2] Parliamentary Act of 1543, quoted in *ibid.*
[3] A. R. Moore, in *Medical Journal of Australia* (1976), vol. 2, no. 18, pp. 736-7.
[4] George Eliot, *Middlemarch* (1871-2), ch. 66.
[5] A. Chekhov, 'House with an Attic' (1890), in *Lady with Lapdog and Other Stories*, trans. David Magarshack (Harmondsworth, Mddx, 1964).

ESSAY 6

[1] George Eliot, *Middlemarch* (1871-2), ch. 66.
[2] R. L. Stevenson, *Underwoods* (1887), pp. i-ii.
[3] Beatrice Webb, *My Apprenticeship* (1926; Harmondsworth, Mddx, 1971), ch. 3.
[4] G. Flaubert, *Madame Bovary* (1857), trans. Alan Russell (Harmondsworth, Mddx, 1972), pt 2, ch. 2.
[5] E. Brontë, 'Lines, October 1837', in *The Complete Poems of Emily Jane Brontë*, ed. C. W. Hatfield (New York, 1941).
[6] Charles Dickens, *Oliver Twist* (1837), ch. 51.
[7] Aldous Huxley, *Brave New World* (1931), foreword.
[8] P. B. Shelley, *The Letters and Prose of Percy Bysshe Shelley*, ed. Roger Ingpen (London, 1909), vol. 5, p. 354.

POSTSCRIPT

Since completing the manuscript of this book I have had the good fortune to join the Society for Health and Human Values, 723 Witherspoon Building, Philadelphia, Pennsylvania, U.S.A., and to gain the benefit of their publications. Two of these earn a very special mention. The first, *Human Values Teaching Programs for Health Professionals* (ed. Thomas K. McElhinney, 3rd ed., 1976), outlines humanistic courses at twenty-nine American universities, all of which share a kinship with the efforts outlined in this book; and the second, *Literature and Medicine* (ed. Joanne Trautmann and Carol Pollard, 1975), is an extensive index of literary works which offer insights into medical and human topics. The latter book has the works grouped and cross-referenced according to period, author, and topic; and outlines a brief synopsis of the medical moments in the work rather than providing the specific extracts.

The author is grateful for permissions granted to quote from the following:

'For a Journey', from *The Railings* by Alan Brownjohn (Macmillan)
The Citadel by A. J. Cronin (the author)
Arrowsmith by Sinclair Lewis (the estate of Sinclair Lewis and Jonathan Cape)
A Very Easy Death by Simone de Beauvoir (Andre Deutsch)
The Immoralist by André Gide (Cassells)
Of Human Bondage by Somerset Maugham (A. P. Watt & Son)
Mrs Dalloway by Virginia Woolf (Hogarth Press)
Brave New World by Aldous Huxley (Mrs Laura Huxley and Chatto & Windus)
Brian's Wife, Jenny's Mum by Gwen Wesson (Dove Publications)
The Magic Faraway Tree by Enid Blyton (Darrell Waters)
The Masters by C. P. Snow (Macmillan)
'My Grandmother Under the Shower', from *Mother I'm Rooted* Kate Jennings (ed.) (Outback Press)
An Old Man Dies by Luise Rinser (S. Fischer Verlag)
'Doctors Warned of Silence on Death', from the *Age* Melbourne (David Syme & Co.)